To Care Enough

To Care Enough

Intervention with Chemically Dependent Colleagues

A Guide for Healthcare and Other Professionals

Linda R. Crosby, M.S.N., R.N.

and

LeClair Bissell, M.D., C.A.C.

Edited by Cyril A. Reilly

A Johnson Institute Book
Professional Series
Minneapolis, MN 1989

A JOHNSON INSTITUTE PROFESSIONAL SERIES BOOK

Published by the Johnson Institute
7151 Metro Blvd., Suite 250
Minneapolis, Minnesota 55435

Library of Congress Cataloging-in-Publication Data

Crosby, Linda R.

　　　To Care Enough

(Professional Series)
Includes bibliographies and index
1. Medical personnel—Substance use. I. Bissell, LeClair. II. Reilly, Cyril A., 1920-   . III. Title. IV. Series: Professional series (Minneapolis, Minn.) [DNLM: 1. Alcoholism—rehabilitation. 2. Health Occupations. 3. Narcotic Dependence—rehabilitation. WM 270 C949t]
RC564.5.M45C76 1989   362.29'08'861   89-7969

ISBN 0-935908-49-8

PRINTED IN THE UNITED STATES OF AMERICA

10 9 8 7 6 5 4 3 2 1

To
the memory of my brother Jay,
whose personal journey
has left footprints on my heart

L.R.C.

For you countless numbers of professionals
who helped, directly and indirectly,
in fighting for treatment rather than
rejection for your colleagues:
If there is now a demand for a book
like this, you helped to create it.
To get the job done, you repeatedly let others
take credit for work that was really yours.
We know, and we thank you.

L.R.C. and LeC.B.

Contents

Acknowledgments

I wish to express my heartfelt gratitude to:

Mom for the special love and care
that nourish my spirit

Dad, Fred, and Faith for the constant support, encouragement,
and love that give me personal strength

Andy Krone, M.D., for helping me to experience reality
with sensitivity, and adversity with a sense of humor

Penny Offer, R.N., for her professional contributions
to the preparation of this manuscript and for encouraging me
when I had doubts

Leo Matti, Executive Director of the Tampa Area Hospital
Council, for believing in
a dream and stepping forth where others dared not tread

The administrators and nursing executives
of the Tampa Area Hospital Council for their active support
of the intervention program
that serves as the foundation of this work

L.R.C.

The authors wish to thank
the Pennsylvania Medical Society, Florida Lawyers
Assistance Program,
Tennessee Nurses Foundation, the Physicians Recovery
Network of Florida,
the California Medical Association, Dr. Thomas Crowley, and
N.U.R.S.E.S. of Colorado
for the material they graciously contributed to this work

Introduction

A Word to Fellow Professionals

If you were presented with information suggesting that a colleague had a problem with alcohol or other drugs, would you know what to do? Would you feel professionally or personally obligated to get involved? Most professionals don't feel prepared to address these questions, because they lack basic knowledge both about chemical dependence* and its devastating personal and professional consequences and about what they can and should do. For many, it's simpler to avoid dealing with the issue. But this allows a progressive disease to get steadily worse, and the end result may be serious physical damage, malpractice, professional exile, and possibly suicide.

The habit of avoiding a chemically dependent colleague's behavior can develop so subtly that we're often unaware of our own need to deny or rationalize. We prefer to see fatigue, overwork, a personal problem, or another medical illness rather than behavior caused by drug use. There are thousands of cases where the physician arrives at the emergency or operating

---

*Editor's Note:
The term "chemical dependence" used throughout this book denotes addiction to and compulsive use of all mind-altering drugs, including alcohol. Although the terms "alcoholism," "substance abuse," "physical and/or emotional dependence," "drug addiction," "drug misuse," and many others are widely used to describe addiction problems, we use the term "chemical dependence" to include dependence on alcohol and all other drugs, regardless of how administered, whether they're illegal, whether physical dependence is a factor, or whether medications are prescribed by one or more physicians, stolen at work, obtained from friends, or bought on the street.

We also use the term "alcohol/other drugs" throughout this book to emphasize that alcohol is a drug—just like cocaine, marijuana, uppers, downers, or any other mind-altering substance. Too often people talk about "alcohol or drugs" or "alcohol and drugs" as if alcohol were somehow different from drugs and in a category by itself. The symptoms of addiction are essentially the same for all these mind-altering drugs, and the need for intervention is just as urgent.

1

room redolent of alcohol and obviously not behaving normally, or where a nurse repeatedly makes alarming medication errors and shows a lack of sound judgment—and yet no action is taken.

Why? Lacking basic knowledge of chemical dependence and its symptoms, and not knowing how to intervene effectively, we colleagues feel helpless. Moreover, we don't want the social stigma attached to alcoholism and other drug addiction, with its traditional suggestion of weakness or moral failure, to hurt one of our own. And it's hard to admit that a beloved friend, a respected colleague, someone prominent in the profession, someone **like us** is chemically dependent. The temptation to dismiss each troublesome event as merely an isolated episode that can be understood and easily explained if seen in context seems irresistible.

Most of us are aware, either from first- or second-hand experience, of incidents where a fellow professional is found to be chemically dependent. In the past, few of these people were given the benefit of a carefully planned and skillfully executed intervention. Even now, many still are lost to their professions by disciplinary action or, ultimately, by illness or death. These losses aren't usually listed as due to alcohol/other drugs and masquerade instead as due to falls, automobile crashes, suicide, liver or cardiac failure, and the like. Unfortunately, we who pride ourselves on our ability to take vigorous action on behalf of patients or clients often become passive spectators when we face chemical dependence in one of our colleagues. We're misled by our own social and personal habits and prejudices as well as by the uncomfortable feelings of powerlessness that come with not knowing how to approach the problem. We fear anger and denial and are further immobilized by the fact that in a world of sophisticated, almost magical, pharmacologic treatments, there's no wonder drug to cure or even subdue more than briefly the symptoms of chemical dependence. And we continually see recidivists who rotate through courts and hospital beds or haunt our offices looking for relief from the medical or social complications of their various addictions. "If he'd only stop drinking..." "She could stop if she really made up her mind to..." "He'll just be back again next month, and we'll have to patch him up again." "This never would have happened if they both weren't on drugs." We hear comments like these in courts, social service agencies, healthcare settings, everywhere, and they reflect our exasperation and lack of knowledge of what chemical dependence is, how it works, and what we can do about it.

We do have an ethical responsibility to our clients or patients to address chemical dependence, both on a professional and a personal level. Most of us are willing to do the right thing, but we aren't sure of exactly how to proceed. Meanwhile, our impaired colleague may be going downhill for months or years. There will be occasional crises, then seeming improvement for a time. Then finally comes the point where we can no longer ignore the problem—we must act.

The good news, though, is that symptoms are present from the onset of the disease and that we can learn to recognize, describe, and identify them and use the data in an early intervention.

"Above all else, to do no harm" is a tenet long embraced by medical professionals. It remains a foundation for what is always an advocacy as well as, at times, a disciplinary process. We have an obligation to know the signs and symptoms of chemical dependence when they appear in a colleague, to understand how we enable our colleagues to continue in their disease, and to know how to do an effective intervention and arrange appropriate treatment. We all know far too many tragic examples of what can happen when colleagues "didn't want to get involved."

Few of us would refuse a colleague who requested help when facing a life crisis. This is, after all, our life's work: We give psychological, spiritual, legal, or medical assistance. Our expertise lies in giving. We do this almost automatically every day for relative strangers who ask for it. Why, then, are we so hesitant to reach out to a colleague? As individuals we can be strong, assertive, and accomplished in our professions, but we tend to avoid situations in which we feel socially uncertain and perhaps personally vulnerable. To try to help a colleague in trouble with alcohol/other drugs means entering uncharted territory. With no maps, we're understandably wary of proceeding. It may seem much safer to ignore or postpone dealing with the problem than to attempt to navigate through it, so we remain on the periphery while our colleagues struggle with their illness and succumb more and more to it. Since they themselves don't ask for help and are usually unable to admit what's wrong, they explain their problems to themselves and to others as due to everything but their use of alcohol/other drugs.

The hope of arresting the disease must come from the outside. Many well-meaning professionals have attempted to help a chemically dependent colleague by "a good heart-to-heart" in hopes that reason alone will help. It may, but usually only temporarily. This approach rarely yields lasting results, since denial is a chief symptom of chemical dependence. These failed appeals to reason, self-discipline, and will power serve only to compound our frustration and to encourage the person in trouble to conceal the problem. To confront a well-established defense system of rationalization, denial, and self-delusion, we need to present indisputable, objective evidence in such a firm but nonthreatening way that the chemically dependent person can really hear it and accept it.

Without outside intervention, some impaired colleagues will continue to function in professional roles, sometimes seemingly successfully, but often increasingly falling below safe standards of practice. Finally their problems may become so blatant that complaints are filed with licensing boards, legal action is taken, or a myriad of other punitive procedures ensue. Disciplinary action by governmental agencies is usually cumbersome and lengthy; it may literally take years to reach a final hearing and a board decision. A license once lost in this fashion is difficult to retrieve, and while the legal process drags on, other colleagues and patients or clients remain at risk.

For many years the myth that alcoholics or other drug addicts couldn't be helped until they themselves wanted help went unchallenged. They had to "hit bottom," the myth said. This simply wasn't and isn't true. There are specific steps to take that can get the person into treatment with an excellent chance that it will work. There may indeed need to be a bottom or a crisis, but bottoms can be raised or a crisis created. There's no need to stand wringing our hands until a disaster occurs. Our challenge is to get help to those who don't believe they need it, don't want it, and therefore rarely seek it on their own. Their families are often equally enmeshed in a denial system of their own that, along with their understandable loyalty conflicts, leaves them paralyzed and incapable of initiating action. Not knowing what help is available, they too seek it in the wrong ways and places or not at all. If they could have done something on their own, there's a good chance they would have done so long before problems became obvious at work.

A knowledgeable colleague may be the only realistic hope for an impaired professional. As colleague and co-worker you possess the reality base, the specific data necessary for action.

This book is your map to using what you've already seen and what you know. It's written especially with the needs of the concerned colleague in mind, one whose concerns are of necessity not the same as those of family members. Even though you may know little or nothing about how bad things may be at your colleague's home or about his or her possible financial or legal difficulties, you have great power. What you say and do may decide whether your colleague will continue to practice his or her chosen profession. The threat of loss of license is an enormous weapon. It must be used fairly and justly, but when needed, it can and should be used. The focus on professional licensure, the risk of its loss (or of disbarment for attorneys), and the threat to the ability to continue in practice is the factor that differentiates professional peer intervention from the traditional family model, since families often must rely on persuasion or the threat of breaking up a marriage or living arrangement. Clearly the focus on licensure is our single most effective leverage when we're dealing with a chemically dependent professional.

In this book we'll cite many examples from the healthcare professions, since these are the professions most familiar to us. But the principles of intervention presented here are much the same for all professions. Like the healthcare professions, the professions of law, psychology, pastoral and other counseling, social work, teaching, and many others usually require licensure or certification. The impaired professional endangers not only himself or herself and family, but also many patients, clients, or students. And the danger is multiplied because licensed professionals are a geographically mobile population who may as a result of their alcohol/other drug use flee to a new state for a "geographical cure" that will also avoid the unpleasant professional consequences of their disease. We must reach these persons before they take matters into their own hands, because flight only postpones the inevitable consequences—consequences that may be grave or even fatal.

You need only two things to reach out and help. The first is **a desire to do so.** The second is **a step-by-step, time-tested plan that shows you exactly how to proceed.** Probably you already have the desire, or you wouldn't have picked up this book. The second you'll understand after you've read it. Yours is a key role. Without your own unique position as colleague and professional to observe the signs and symptoms visible only to you, there may not be enough significant data for the intervention. Family members may be helpless or indifferent; they can rarely judge what's happening at work. Remember, too, that the principles of intervention you learn from this book will be helpful in intervening not only with a colleague but also with other chemically dependent people you may well meet in your professional practice.

Intervening isn't comfortable or easy. You'll be tempted to cut corners or follow only a few of our suggestions. Please don't. If something doesn't make sense to you, check it out with others who are skilled in these matters before deciding to ignore it and plunge in semi-prepared. The major reason why colleagues sometimes fail despite their sincere and well-meaning attempts is that they haven't taken the time and trouble to approach the situation properly. To feel that these things rarely work is often a mistaken attempt to blame the victim or the situation rather than the professionalism of the intervenors. Both authors have had the experience of approaching an intervention ill prepared. As we look back on those incidents both of us wish that someone had written down for us what we're telling you in this book. Learning about intervention and actually doing one may be one of the most challenging tasks you'll ever undertake, but it may also be one of the most rewarding. Your knowledge and your willingness to help a colleague may save both a career and a life— perhaps many careers, many lives. Don't waste your opportunity.

Part I

Chemical Dependence and Intervention:
The Problem, the Solution

Chapter 1

Understanding the Problem of Chemical Dependence

If you have an inquiring mind, you may be asking, "Just how big a problem is chemical dependence in the professions?" Frankly, no one can give us exact figures, but even conservative estimates are sobering (no pun intended). The following discussion explains why.

Chemical Dependence in the Professions: How Big a Problem?

Trying to answer how big the problem is soon reveals that we need to break it down into several questions, which we'll consider in turn:
• What percentage of professionals are chemically dependent?
• Why can't we predict who will become chemically dependent?
• Are there behaviors and effects of compulsive alcohol/other drug use that enable us to recognize it so we can do an early intervention?
• If there are clear indicators of compulsive alcohol/other drug use, why do we often fail to recognize them?

What Percentage of Professionals Are Chemically Dependent?

When one of us presented a proposal to a group of hospital administrators to fund a community-wide intervention program for nurses, their first question was "How many nurses are we actually talking about?"—definitely a concern if this venture was to be cost-effective. When we mentioned the estimated

20% reported in some of the literature, there was understandable skepticism, so we agreed to figure only 10%. Even so, that meant that with 4000 licensed nurses in that county alone, 400 might be in trouble with alcohol/other drugs. Realizing that even one impaired nurse could create a huge liability, the group funded the program.

The truth is that we still have no accurate statistics of the percentage of professionals afflicted with the disease: social workers, counselors, psychologists, priests, nuns, attorneys, doctors, nurses, teachers, dentists, veterinarians, pharmacists, airline pilots, and others. Literature on this subject offers guesses of anywhere from 9% to 20%, and treatment experts think that the truth lies with the larger estimates, probably somewhere between 10% and 15%.

Why we have no accurate data is simple. First, if you were asked to count the number of Kelly clamps, McGill forceps, depositions, incompetency papers, or Schedule II drugs in a given place but you had no idea of what those items were or how to recognize them, would you expect to do a good job of it? Hardly. But that's just the trouble with sizing up accurately how many professionals are chemically dependent: Many people who deal day after day with such professionals and who might be expected to recognize their condition and report it to someone who can help don't really know what chemical dependence is or how to recognize it. And so the records remain incomplete.

Secondly, when impaired professionals have undergone disciplinary action by licensing boards for such violations as unprofessional conduct, negligence, improper handling of controlled drugs, or diversion of controlled drugs for personal use, these disciplinary actions are recorded only under the broad, vague category of violation and don't always specify whether alcohol/other drugs were involved.

Thirdly, not all who are in trouble are caught or, even when they are, reported.

Fourthly, not all who are reported are found guilty, even when they are. Even though it's still common to fire such persons, authorities often cite some other reason for the firing. Why? Explanations often given are "lack of proof," fear of litigation, fear of anger and retaliation, and a common "let-someone-else-deal-with-it" attitude. Establishing that someone has a problem with alcohol or prescription drugs is even more difficult than in the case of controlled drugs, because controlled drugs are often stolen on the job and therefore leave a detectable paper trail. But even among the controlled drugs, marijuana and cocaine are usually bought on the street, so there's hardly ever any written record to indicate their purchase or use. Where persons with alcohol/other drug problems are fired but aren't reported because another reason has been given for their dismissal, they often move on to practice in different locations, even in different states. In the new area there will of course be no record of problems with licensing boards.

Despite our admitted lack of accurate figures on the numbers of chemically impaired professionals, it's clear that the situation is serious. Various state agency reports of completed disciplinary actions show that a clear majority of all disbarments and revocations of medical, pharmacy, physician assistant, and nursing licenses are related to alcohol/other drug use. Still, only a small percentage of such cases ever get reported, and states and disciplines vary widely in the degree to which they assume responsibility for regulating professionals. (Psychologists and social workers are more likely to face charges for sexual misbehavior with their patients and clients than for alcohol/other drug problems. But that's no reason to believe they have fewer problems with them than other professionals do or even that some of the sexual acting out isn't associated with alcohol/other drug problems.)

Another indication that we're dealing with a serious problem is that almost every major professional association has a policy statement about alcohol/other drug use, and many also have state-level programs for assisting their members. However, even if only a few judges, dentists, teachers, clergy, nurses, physicians, dentists, or pharmacists were impaired, the situation would still call for action. We know that any trusted professional who's chemically dependent can do immeasurable harm, and that fact demands our full attention and early commitment to help. Here are two examples.

A nurse working on a chemotherapy unit was suspected of diverting Demerol (a powerful synthetic narcotic), but the hospital administration felt it lacked adequate documentation to take action. Several months later she made five gross errors on a single shift: She administered two wrong medications, one of them chemotherapy, administered the wrong blood plasma, administered a double dose of narcotic to a patient, then left the unit unattended for half an hour. Her supervisors were waiting for proof as her disease progressed and the danger mounted! Unfortunately, intervention wasn't initiated until these errors were discovered and patients had been hurt.

It's not surprising that her supervisors, when finally comparing notes, could readily identify examples of a gradual decline in level of performance over several months, abrupt mood swings, and "forgetfulness" that had resulted in omitting medication and treatment. By the time her performance was blatantly impaired, she had progressed to an advanced stage of chemical dependence and was walking a tightrope, endangering her own life and that of her patients. During her first weeks of treatment, she required intensive medical management of her detoxification because of her prolonged use of high dosages of narcotics, sedatives, and cocaine. During the months before her treatment, she had been unable to maintain her home and had been evicted. She was being divorced by her husband, who had left some time before and was attempting to gain custody of their child.

Again, a skillful and well-loved surgeon was known to his colleagues as a heavy drinker. They knew that he had left his wife and set up housekeeping with another woman in the back room of his office. For a time his work performance was adequate, and there were no reports of any harm to patients. But as new techniques developed in his field, he opted not to learn them and instead limited his work to procedures that were familiar, safe, and almost automatic. He became increasingly withdrawn socially, stopped editing and writing for journals, refused election to office in professional societies. What he did he did well enough, but he did less and less, a phenomenon often referred to as "job shrinkage." While there were no obvious crises, people knew him less and less well, and gradually began to feel that in some unnamed way they just didn't trust him quite as they had before. If he ever did make a major error in patient care, we're still not aware of it. But very late one evening he was killed driving alone on the turnpike. He was drunk. None of us had made any attempt to reach out to him, but some of us still miss him and grieve that we never even tried.

Unfortunately, these aren't isolated examples of waiting until things have reached the crisis point or caused a tragedy. It happens in every profession and will continue until we insist on change.

Why Can't We Predict Chemical Dependence?

The answer is easy: because there simply are no reliable ways to predict who will become chemically dependent. There's no typical personality, no set of physical attributes, just as there's no area of practice, no setting or career that's immune. A nun with a master's degree and a nursing background worked as a hospital administrator. She was also an addict. The disease crosses all sociological, ethnic, professional, and geographic borders, so it's impossible to identify an addict in any given group unless the person shows signs and symptoms of the disease. Even though chemical dependence is familial, it's still impossible to predict which persons in a high-risk family will develop problems.

Studies of professionals now in recovery indicate that they were generally well regarded by their colleagues, had been high academic achievers, and were frequently quite accomplished in their fields. They weren't the losers or even borderline performers. Often they were the "doers," talented persons respected by colleagues and loved by clients or patients. Their contributions to their fields of practice were acknowledged time after time by colleagues, by friends who later exclaimed, "I can't believe it," "Not so-and-so, the best nurse [doctor, young priest, or lawyer] we have," "She's much too bright," or "It's got to be a mistake!" However, the real mistake is to believe it's a mistake! Academic prowess and professional accomplishments don't ward off illness.

Are There Reliable Signs of Chemical Dependence?

Despite the fact that there are no **easily applied, objective measures** to yield a positive or negative diagnosis unless one does a drug screen, observes old and new needle "tracks" over the veins, or can persuade a colleague to fill out an alcohol/other drug use assessment test with full candor, there nevertheless are recognizable behaviors and visible effects of compulsive alcohol/other drug use that we **can** identify, even early on in the process, that provide us with probable and therefore sufficient cause for intervention.

Perhaps the most critical component of this identification is knowing the performance baseline from which a person has normally functioned. When behavior and practice clearly move **away** from this normal performance baseline, it indicates some sort of problem. We're all entitled to have an occasional bad day, but it's different when one has increasingly frequent bad days. We don't usually suspect a colleague of alcohol/other drug use because he or she sometimes appears irritable, argumentative, even drowsy or withdrawn, misses a filing date, or once in a while forgets to write orders, administer medications, change intravenous fluids, or order pre-op medications. Mistakes are human. But mistakes that happen with increasing frequency are something else again. Without actually confirming our assumptions, we at first attribute many of these changes to overwork, to busy schedules, or to a problem at home. But when these changes cease to be rare and isolated episodes, we begin to see **patterns** that are common indicators of chemical dependence. What we finally notice is usually only the tip of the iceberg, because professionals struggle to maintain their professional standards and continue functioning for a long time in spite of their active addictions before they reach a point of deterioration that's impossible to ignore. (One librarian said that the closest she had ever come to heroism was getting to work on time in spite of the almost constant nausea and headache that were part of her daily morning hangovers.)

Why Don't We Recognize Clear Signs?

Simply put, once we know and acknowledge that we know, we may have to get involved. It's much safer and simpler not to know! Involvement with a chemically dependent colleague involves risk. Our fears surface when we're faced with the "what ifs": "What if I'm wrong?" "What if he denies it?" "What if she threatens to sue?" And, probably the worst fear, if the people are close to us, "What if they get angry and reject me?" "They" may include the mutual friends and co-workers who may side with the chemically dependent person, not with the would-be helper.

Of course we're not always aware of these fears. They usually arrive almost immediately, dressed in familiar rationalizations that deter us from action. "This would be a bad time to do anything, with everyone else who can be spared already on vacation for August." "It's probably just a temporary situation." "This is simply the result of overwork or stress. It'll be better when things ease up." "He's seeing a therapist who'll take care of it. Meddling with someone in treatment just isn't done." (One alcoholic psychoanalyst, now long sober, reports drinking throughout her training at a world-famous analytic institute, even drinking while seeing her patients. She thoughtfully brought soft drinks to the children's sessions so they wouldn't feel left out. This was known to several colleagues, all of whom deferred to the training analyst, who they assumed would take care of the matter. They evidently said nothing to the training analyst, who, in fact, never once mentioned drinking as a problem or paid attention to the patient's half-hearted attempts to bring it up.) It's these common fears of facing anger or being attacked by one's colleagues for being a whistle blower, and reluctance to get involved in a potentially sticky situation that, combined with old myths and attitudes and our own lack of experience, prevent us from becoming first-line advocates for our colleagues.

Defining and Understanding Chemical Dependence

Before we can help our colleague who's suffering from chemical dependence, we need to understand what it is and how it works.

Chemical dependence as defined by Vernon Johnson is a **primary, progressive, chronic disease that is ultimately fatal if not treated.** Probably the most important thing for us to understand as helping professionals is that it's a primary disease—that is, not a symptom of something else. Like any other primary disease, it must be addressed in its own right. It's perfectly true that many chemically dependent people are suffering from marital discord, agonized by a favorite child's own drug problem, or plagued by depression, accidents, or financial and medical woes, but these are all too often not the causes of alcohol/other drug use but the results of it. Of course alcoholics and other addicts can have other problems as well. Being alcoholic is obviously no guarantee that pregnancy, appendicitis, or mental illness may not also be present and warrant attention, but the alcohol use still must be addressed in its own right. These other matters are important but separate issues.

To understand chemical dependence, we must look at the interaction between the alcohol/other drug and the person. Most of us have been introduced to some drug: probably alcohol, or perhaps an amphetamine to help us study for an exam, perhaps a little smoking (or a lot). Most of us would probably say the experience induced a pleasant feeling, perhaps a carefree attitude and mild euphoria. After all, we wouldn't drink or use more than a few times if the experience weren't pleasant. Socially, we develop our own patterns of drinking, for instance, and learn what effects alcohol has on us in different situations. For example, if a drink on an empty stomach leads to feeling light-headed, we usually solve the problem by eating something first, drinking more slowly, or drinking less. We learn how many drinks we can tolerate without becoming embarrassingly drunk or suffering painful hangovers. One factor remains constant: The feeling induced by the alcohol is **pleasurable**.

In contrast to what we've just described, the person who's **dependent** on alcohol or another drug loses the ability to predict its effects, to stop while ahead of the game, and to limit consumption predictably. As one uses more of the drug, tolerance builds, and more of it is required to achieve that same pleasant effect, so one increases the amount in an attempt to feel good.

Initially this poses few problems; and many users, particularly young male drinkers, gain status from their ability to down large quantities and still appear unaffected. We should emphasize that professionals typically don't at first use drugs other than alcohol, marijuana, or cocaine just to get "high." More frequently they're attempting to stay awake in spite of fatigue or to manage physical or psychogenic pain. This is important in understanding what happens at the onset of the disease. No one consciously sets out to become addicted to alcohol/other drugs. People who later become addicts use drugs much as everyone else uses them: to feel a little less tense, to be a little less shy, a little more comfortable, a bit more relaxed, to sleep or to stay awake, or because others are using and it seems the socially correct thing to do. To resist a drink at a wedding, at Mardi Gras, on New Year's Eve or Saint

Patrick's Day can give an older adult the same sort of experience of peer pressure that a college student of the sixties faced when it seemed everyone was smoking marijuana.

Three Elements of Fully Developed Chemical Dependence

While the causes of chemical dependence still aren't fully understood, significant research supports a strong genetic element as well as social and individual personality influences that are important in the differing degrees of illness of different persons. Whatever those causes are, fully developed chemical dependence has three elements: 1) loss of predictability, 2) compulsive use, and 3) continued use in spite of adverse consequences. Notice, there's no mention of diagnosing the disease by observing withdrawal symptoms (to detect physical dependence) or by measuring the quantity, frequency, and duration of use. Healthcare and other professionals have placed too much emphasis on issues of quantity and frequency, on physical dependence, or on the belief that to be an alcoholic, for instance, one has to drink until drunk on every drinking occasion or to remain drunk a majority of the waking hours, or that to be addicted to other drugs one must have severe withdrawal symptoms when the drugs are removed. "Drugs," of course, popularly refers to those that are controlled or illegal or that haven't been prescribed by a physician. Oddly enough, alcohol, our nation's most devastating drug, is rarely referred to as a drug. Sound familiar?

Let's expand a bit on the editor's note given in the Introduction. The reason for using the admittedly clumsy term "chemical dependence" is to include within it problems with **all** mind-altering drugs that have the potential of creating dependence. Using this term reflects an attempt to be more inclusive than if only the word "drugs" were used and the reader were allowed to think only in terms of opiates. Addiction doesn't refer to physical dependence alone, nor does it refer exclusively to illicit drugs. For healthcare professionals, common drugs such as the benzodiazepines (Valium, Librium), sedative hypnotics (Nembutal, Placidyl), amphetamines (Dexedrine, Benzedrine), or alcohol are fully as likely to pose problems as the drugs that are more upsetting to the public (cocaine, heroin, marijuana). Addiction potential and toxicity aren't well measured by whether a drug is illegal. Quantity used and legal status are of interest, but the crucial question is what the drug is doing to the person and what he or she is prepared to lose rather than give it up. When a person is willing to risk the safety of children, the love and respect of spouse and colleagues, the ability to practice a valued profession, even at times the physical freedom to avoid jail, but can't or won't stop using, it makes little

16

difference whether the disasters occur daily or only once a week or whether there's a demonstrable withdrawal state as the person becomes drug-free. Most alcoholics and other addicts are in some control of their use most of the time, or it wouldn't be so easy for them to explain away to themselves, even more than to others, the consequences they accept rather than stop.

Let's look now at each of the three elements of fully developed chemical dependence.

Loss of Predictability. Loss of predictability refers to the fact that a chemically dependent person has lost the ability to predict two things: how much alcohol or other drugs he or she will use on a given occasion, and what the effects of that use will be. This loss of predictability is obviously a serious matter, since the chemical dependent (to say nothing of family, friends, employers, and possibly many others whose safety and perhaps their very lives depend on this person) has no way of knowing what terrible things might happen as the result of any drinking or using episode.

A frequent companion of loss of predictability is the blackout. A blackout is often confused with passing out. But the two aren't the same, even though a person using alcohol/other drugs can pass out **during** a blackout. Passing out means unconsciousness: The person appears to fall asleep abruptly. A blackout is different and usually has nothing to do with falling asleep. It's drug-induced amnesia: a period of seconds, minutes, hours, perhaps days during which the person is awake and active but later remembers nothing about the events that took place. During this time, the person may or, amazingly, may **not** appear intoxicated. In fact, he or she might seem quite normal, though usually high.

Blackouts can go unnoticed by others. Serious mishaps (such as auto accidents, arrests for driving under the influence, or serious omissions in job performance) may occur during the blackout. Sometimes the behavior seems entirely normal to others, but for the one experiencing the blackout, a piece of the day or evening is missing. One head nurse called her unit at six in the morning to say that she was ill, wouldn't be in to work, and that a replacement should be called in. This was done. Just before eight o'clock the head nurse arrived as usual, every hair in place and smelling of breath mints, quite puzzled as to why her staff was surprised to see her. The episode either wasn't reported or was misunderstood. (Three years later, police found this same nurse intoxicated and barricaded in her apartment, where she had been hallucinating and smashing plates and furniture.) One episode of this kind would probably make most of us resolve never to repeat the experience, a promise we'd be able to make to ourselves and keep. The chemically dependent person, though, may make that promise to self but be unable to honor it and within a few hours may again have a drink, pill bottle, or syringe in hand.

Frequent blackouts are such a reliable sign of chemical dependence that their presence is almost the only evidence we need in order to know that that person is chemically dependent. But the **absence** of blackouts is no sign that the person **isn't** chemically dependent, because not all chemical dependents experience blackouts (probably some 15% don't).

Loss of predictability, then, is even a surer sign of chemical dependence than blackouts are. Even the onset of loss of predictability is unpredictable; it may occur early or late after one begins drinking/using; it may come before or after one starts having blackouts (or, as we've mentioned, may happen even if blackouts never occur). In short, it's such a reliable indicator of chemical dependence that we can almost define a chemical dependent as a person who has lost the ability to predict on a given drinking/using occasion how much he or she will drink/use (or, if the person hasn't been using lately, when the use will resume) or to predict what the effects will be.

Compulsive Use. Many chemically dependent healthcare professionals know that taking drugs from the narcotics supply is wrong, and they don't want to continue this behavior, but they can't stop it. We hear, "Every day I said I'm not going to do this again, even while I was opening the narcotics cabinet." With loss of control over the illness comes a dilemma. These people know they're violating the law and the ethical foundations of their profession, but just knowing isn't enough. The professional rapidly becomes engulfed in guilt and concealment. This in turn increases the need both to avoid additional problems and to get drug-induced relief. If the drug of choice is a stolen controlled drug, or if one is sneaking out to visit a crack dealer more and more regularly, the fear and self-loathing increase even more because one feels like an outlaw. If it's alcohol, the drinker is more likely to feel inadequate or lacking in will power, since he or she can no longer do successfully what everyone else seems able to do. Facing these seemingly insoluble problems, however, almost all chemically dependent people somehow manage to believe that something external will change and that they'll regain the ability to stop using or to use only in moderation.

Some of Alcoholics Anonymous' old hands are fond of saying that once a cucumber becomes a pickle, it can never go back to being a cucumber. True enough. Fortunately, most of us realize that once an opiate addict starts mainlining, he or she probably won't be able to return to Saturday night "chipping" (skin popping). Most of us would think twice before urging a former heavy smoker to return to only two or three cigarettes after dinner. But it's equally silly to encourage an alcoholic to drink only a little, although sometimes those of us who point this out are called rigid and moralistic. It would indeed be easier to offer addicts goals other than abstinence, just as it would be nice to offer young diabetics something other than a lifelong need for insulin. But life dictates otherwise. We mustn't nourish unrealistic expectations or distort the truth because it's unpleasant. Once a colleague is seriously in trouble with alcohol/other drugs, we must find a way to help that person stop and stay stopped, not just from the drug that has been the major problem but from all other mind-altering drugs as well.

Once our chemically dependent colleagues are solidly enmeshed in their addictions, they usually can't stop permanently by themselves. Without the drug, life is too much; and to complicate matters, physical dependence may now have appeared. Feeling unable to manage without it, they'll do whatever it takes to obtain it. For many, securing the drug becomes the primary focus of their life, particularly when it must be obtained illegally. This may require large amounts of time, money, and energy. They may lose sight of all else around them until they have a supply. They need it to survive.

Since one is rarely able to stop this process without treatment, there usually must be a well-planned intervention, and the sooner the better.

Continued Use in Spite of Adverse Consequences. Ultimately, chemically dependent people seem to become fused with their drug of choice. They develop such a narrowly focused view of the world that only the drug really matters. Family, friends, and profession fade into the periphery. Many describe this condition as "having a love relationship with the drug." One attorney, a regular cocaine user, was asked which seemed more important to him, his drug or sex. Almost condescendingly, he answered, "Cocaine is sex!" Within three months after that his job, wife, house, and car were gone, and he said, "It all went up my nose."

The feelings and behavior of chemically dependent persons parallel those of infatuation: Much energy is spent thinking about and fantasizing about the drug and what it will do. Adverse consequences erupt in many different areas of their lives, probably first at home. They become increasingly withdrawn and give less and less time and attention to family matters; they may become unpredictable, paranoid, and explosive, sometimes even violent. The upset this causes in family relationships only increases the need for relief, and they drift farther and farther from those they love. Many suffer the loss of their families long before receiving help, even if the families remain present as virtual strangers under the same roof. As important as significant others are, even the threat of losing them is often not enough to force an admission that anything is amiss, much less that they need help or will accept it.

There are other consequences such as acting inappropriately at social gatherings or getting into arguments and fights. Estrangement from the local community and its activities may follow, perhaps helped along by a local newspaper account of a Driving While Intoxicated (DWI) or other arrest.

But none of these consequences alone usually has enough impact to stop the drinking or using more than briefly. Rather, one hears, "I shouldn't have driven that night," "It was mixing drinks that did me in," "My wife is getting on my case, so I'll cut down a little," or "I'll just not drink at the club with that bunch anymore." Chemical dependents still believe they can **control** their alcohol/other drug use. They may indeed cut down or even abstain entirely for a while, but one thing is predictable: Without treatment or a serious commitment to participate in a self-help group such as Alcoholics Anonymous (A.A.), Narcotics Anonymous (N.A.), or Cocaine Anonymous (C.A.), most will return to the old patterns, whether it happens within a week, a month, or even a year or more. Significant symptoms may not appear at work until a late stage of the disease. Simply put, the job is usually the last thing to go. That doesn't mean that it doesn't go, however. One's professional identity may even support the delusion of normalcy in the face of other consequences. "I still have my practice, my license, my profession." "Things can't be that bad; I still have my work. I'll straighten myself out." "I'm good at what I do. I can always start over and do it somewhere else."

Unfortunately, the denial system so typical of chemical dependence is characterized by a myriad of delusions that reinforce the belief that the problem is under control. For some persons the professional identity (license) becomes the single most treasured possession, the undeniable proof that they're really all right even though everything else is crumbling. No wonder any threat to it gets their attention. "But I'm a doctor," "I'm a lawyer," "I'm a nurse. This can't have happened to me." So they struggle to maintain their delusions even in the face of overwhelming contradictory evidence. Even when they're finally threatened with disbarment, loss of license, and subsequent loss of livelihood, it's sometimes not enough to convince them that they need help. Many have actually undergone disciplinary proceedings by licensing boards and yet have never connected the consequences with their alcohol/other drug use. Everyone and everything else is to blame!

Sincere in their delusion that the alcohol/other drug use hasn't created the problems, they rationalize, deny, and project the blame onto others and onto circumstances. All the warnings and threats from licensing boards may not break this denial. Since drugs are **not** the problem, they continue to use.

Profession-Specific Issues

Besides being swayed by the same factors that move the general population toward chemical dependence, members of many professions are exposed to certain additional factors precisely because they belong to that profession—what we can call profession-specific problems. Healthcare professionals are a case in point. Their twin demons are so-called "pharmacologic optimism" (excessive faith in medications) and easy access to mind-altering drugs. They have a sophisticated knowledge of drug actions, interactions, and therapeutic dosages and depend on this knowledge to alleviate suffering and promote wellness. They also have great faith in the ability of intellect and information to protect them. Much of their "medical model" is based on rapid chemo-therapeutic interventions. They have a drug for almost every possible clinical situation and feel competent and assured when giving it. They need only look at standard orders on a patient chart to realize how many of the orders are for medications. Even if the doctor fails to prescribe "something for every ill," the nurse often will solicit the orders from the doctor. Drugs are the tools of the trade; giving them is something healthcare people can actually **do** for patients that requires very little time. And they usually work!

Practitioners are rewarded for their actions. The patient feels better, looks better, and often expresses gratitude for the relief. Imagine the quantity of medications healthcare people prescribe, administer, dispense, or see used in a typical day. That's a lot of positive reinforcement! Practitioners begin to feel omnipotent in dealing with medications. They know and understand them far too well to fear them. Trusting in drugs, which they call "medications," becomes second nature.

When healthcare professionals find themselves in need of medical treatment or relief of pain, they frequently prescribe for themselves whatever is on the shelf in a bathroom cabinet or available in the office or pharmacy and feel quite comfortable in doing so. After all, why bother a colleague unnecessarily to do the identical prescribing? The next step is simply to borrow a medication from the patient stock, whether it's an antibiotic, muscle relaxant, or pain reliever. No one would say to a colleague, "No, you can't have Darvocet from the stock, even if you're busy, unless you get someone else to prescribe it and then put the prescription through the pharmacy." How silly! Who would struggle through eight hours with a pounding headache?

We mention this apparently acceptable behavior for two reasons. First, many healthcare professionals have developed double standards for their practice. Second, this behavior is really no different from borrowing from the patient stock a dose of any drug for anyone else. As professionals become comfortable with self-medicating and there's no negative consequence, there's no obstacle to doing it regularly. This is common behavior in many hospitals. After all, professionals with too much to do shouldn't waste their own time and everyone else's going through meaningless formalities.

Somewhere in that established pattern is added the belief "I won't keep working well if I don't get some relief" or "I can't go home, they need me here," and this belief reinforces the process. So it's a short step from mild analgesics to the narcotic box when one needs immediate relief. After all, it's only for this one occasion, and it's readily available on the medication cart. The only difference is that one has to sign for it. Furthermore, when a patient is administered a narcotic but needs only half of what's in the syringe, the rest would normally (according to federal regulations) be discarded. Since no one will use it anyway and some "relief" is needed now, the first self-injection occurs. At the time, it's "only going to happen once." Interestingly, many nurses say that their first dose of a narcotic taken for relief from pain came from a dose that otherwise would have been "wasted." Some indeed may have had quite real physical pain, but many were instead suffering emotional distress and disequilibrium.

This same story is reported for oral narcotics such as Tylox, Percodan, Tylenol #3, or Florinal. The first self-administered dose, no matter how innocent it appears at the time, often begins the progressive illness of chemical dependence. Healthcare professionals have become addicted to pain relievers received after undergoing surgical procedures and dental work. A nurse undergoing an outpatient gynecologic procedure was given Demerol as a pre-operative medication and remembered distinctly the floating feeling and how good it felt. Several months later when going through a painful divorce and custody battle, she was working in a pediatric unit. A child had been ordered to receive Demerol, but the amount actually needed was minute, so she took the rest home with her to take after work. This initiated a daily pattern that persisted for six months. She passed out several times in the bathroom while injecting, and experienced blackouts while on duty, but she wasn't confronted until very late in her addiction.

The interaction of the drug and the individual involves many elements, and each person reacts uniquely to a given drug. Although people don't necessarily become addicted to a certain drug, **they can become addicted to the feeling it produces** and will seek out the same or similar drugs to get that feeling or something approximating it. If narcotics were controlled more stringently, would there be less chemical dependence? Probably not, since the feeling sought could still be found through alcohol/other drugs. People now in recovery have a saying, "If you can't be near the drug you love, you love the drug you're near." Most chemically dependent people are polydrug users;

even those identified as pure alcoholics use tranquilizers and sedatives at times. The process is the same, no matter which drug is used. Healthcare professionals do know better when it comes to prescribing medications, but often they don't realize that they themselves can be seduced as easily as anyone else and that they may be even harder to warn and convince because of their own expertise with drugs.

The Emotional Syndrome of Chemical Dependence

Chemical dependence, as we've briefly noted, involves the interaction of personality, genetics, environment, and social influences. But to describe this disease fully, we must look specifically at its emotional effects.

Vernon Johnson has described four stages in the emotional as distinguished from the merely physical syndrome of chemical dependence: 1) learning the mood swing, 2) seeking the mood swing, 3) harmful dependence, and 4) drinking/using to feel normal again.* The underlying premise of Johnson's model is that everyone normally experiences various emotions, ranging from painful ones to euphoria, depending on interactions with other people and one's environment. One's position on the continuum varies throughout any given day, depending on individual emotional experiences. However, most people fall within a median range on this continuum—a range we call normal.

Emotional Continuum

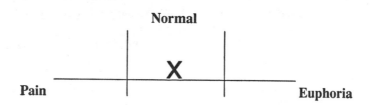

* For more detailed descriptions read *Intervention: How to Help Someone Who Doesn't Want Help* by Vernon E. Johnson, D.D. (Minneapolis: Johnson Institute, 1986).

Let's discuss these four stages.

1. Learning the Mood Swing

We said earlier that the drug induced a pleasurable feeling. This is another way of describing the first stage of the emotional development of dependence: learning the mood swing. When people who later become chemically dependent take their first drink or other drug, they discover, though perhaps not till after a few false starts, that it's definitely a pleasant experience. They feel better, which means the drug has moved them along the continuum toward the euphoric end. This doesn't mean they're necessarily high from one drink or one joint, but the pleasurable feeling does reinforce repeating the experience. If one dose of a drug made them feel good, two might be even better.

Emotional Continuum, Stage 1

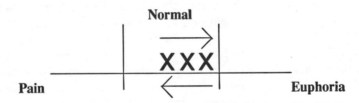

However, in this first stage when the drug wears off, users return to a normal feeling state. But they've learned that a certain amount of a drug will induce a very pleasant emotional state, and they begin to look forward to repeating the experience. Initially they may use alcohol/other drugs only to relax after work, or to unwind socially and feel less inhibited, but they're sure it will always achieve the desired result. So they're beginning to develop a relationship with the drug. Remember the analogy of "having a love relationship with a drug"? A person who's feeling this strong pull is ready to move into Stage 2.

2. Seeking the Mood Swing

As this stage develops, users rely heavily on the drug to ward off unpleasant feelings, fatigue, or worries and begin to use it more regularly. Despite the fact that many persons occasionally drink or use too much, they may remain in Stage 2 and never suffer adverse consequences. They may even get drunk or high on occasion, but usually the worst price they pay is a minor embarrassment or a hangover before the body returns to normal. An important point is that they still do return to the normal range of the emotional continuum after using the drug.

Stage 2 may be as short as a few weeks for some and years for others. There are no absolute predictors of exactly when people will move into Stage 3: harmful dependence. This is one of the least understood aspects of the disease. However, while users remain in Stage 2 the behavior related to the use is changing gradually. There's now increasing anticipation of using the drug, and excessive use may be more frequent. As the need for the drug increases, so usually does the tolerance. In other words, it now takes more than two drinks, one joint, two pills, one line to get the same relief or high. This tolerance initiates a compulsion to have access to enough of the drug. Users now begin to plan how and where to use or to get enough of it to make them feel the way they want to feel. For some, this planning itself becomes an adventure in anticipation. They arrange their schedules so that nothing interferes with their "date with the drug." Early in this stage they may attempt to establish controls for themselves as to when they may drink or use. This gives them a sense of mastery over the alcohol/other drug. They may decide to drink only beer, only wine, only after five o'clock, or to use cocaine only on weekends, or only with certain friends. However, as tolerance and dependence build, they become increasingly unable to predict their own patterns or amounts of use. For some professionals there's a taboo on drinking before work or at lunch if one is working in the afternoon. This is an obvious consideration for healthcare and other professionals, yet many progress to using before work, then to using at work. This can be such a gradual process that one isn't consciously aware of violating his or her own rules for use.

Emotional Continuum, Stage 2

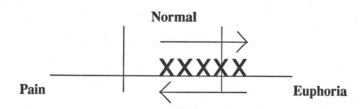

Some rely on others to keep matters under control, and this can be partially successful, at least for a while. Several women religious, all of them nurses or educators, describe the changes during the seventies when, free of religious garb (and hence of easy recognition), they were able to go into many previously forbidden places and for the first time make their own decisions about drinking. Before that, a superior had controlled the supply, doling it out only on special occasions or in small amounts. Now, with no experience in setting their own limits and with much less external structure to use as a substitute, some got into trouble very quickly. The changes didn't cause their alcoholism any more than the old system had been able to prevent it altogether, but having someone else in charge—be it a religious superior, a managing spouse, or even "Mother Army"—can slow it down for a time.

Obtaining a desired drug, even for healthcare professionals, soon becomes a challenge. Sometimes the drug is available in the hospital, but users must find ways to take it without arousing suspicion. It's not uncommon to hear chemically dependent nurses or doctors say, "Every day when I went to work, I had to figure a way to get the Demerol. Once I had it in my pocket I knew everything would be all right." It's important to note (as we did earlier in passing) that these people usually aren't just seeking pleasure. They're usually attempting to cope with emotional or physical situations that they see as stressful and as interfering with their ability to perform professionally. Often from the very beginning they see the use as "self-medication" for a temporary problem—nothing more. They've already experienced the desired effect. They know about the mood swing and have effectively learned that alcohol or another drug does in fact appear to alleviate the problem. The need for it is now increasing, and professionals will violate personal and professional ethical standards to obtain it, through fraud and tampering with narcotic and patient records or borrowing from clients' funds if necessary. But despite the fact that users need more of the drug, need it more frequently, and begin to plan situations for using it, they still may have suffered no serious adverse emotional consequences. They're still able to return to a normal feeling state when they stop using.

3. Harmful Dependence

When users move into Stage 3 of the disease, they no longer merely return to normal on the feeling continuum but gradually move into the pain range. In other words, they can't bounce back with impunity from the use; they experience real emotional discomfort after the alcohol/other drug use. They rebound into exactly the feeling state the drug was taken to change, but now it's even worse. Even though, for example, one took alcohol or tranquilizers in order to feel less tense and more relaxed, now there's more anxiety and tension than before. Or if one took cocaine or amphetamines to boost confidence and energy and get rid of depression, one is now even more depressed and listless.

Emotional Continuum, Stage 3

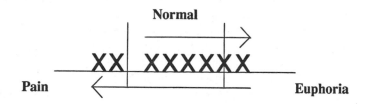

Frequently Stage 3 users act inappropriately, become argumentative and disruptive while using, and then are faced with the memory of that behavior the next day. They may be embarrassed and remorseful but quickly decide that the reason for the misbehavior was their drinking on an empty stomach, putting a drink on top of an antihistamine, using too strong a dose of a drug, not getting enough sleep, or being upset because someone provoked them. People who are becoming increasingly chemically dependent rarely consciously see their using the drug as the problem. Instead they point to the special circumstances surrounding the use. They spend great energy rationalizing the "how" of the event rather than the "why," which of course is the drug itself. As the process continues, behaviors become more unpredictable, even bizarre at times, and this creates heavy pressure on users' self-esteem. They remain quite sincerely unaware that the drug is the cause of the problem, so they must blame either themselves for their "bad temper" or someone else's "bad temper" or something other than the alcohol/other drug use for causing the problem.

This becomes a vicious cycle in the harmful-dependence stage: excessive use, inappropriate behavior, accusation of those closest and most easily available as scapegoats, self-blame, and guilt. The emotional cost and the pain of the chemical dependence increase. Progressively, ego strength deteriorates, and users try to get relief through more of the drug. In the past it rarely failed to deliver the desired change of feeling, but now the beginning isn't a normal feeling state but rather a painful and anxious one. It isn't hard to understand that to move from the least comfortable end of the spectrum to the euphoric end takes greater and greater amounts of the drug and more frequent use.

As the now-serious dependence becomes more extreme, many areas of users' lives are affected—intimate relationships usually first, work only later. Again, chemical dependents rationalize that "people, places, and things" have caused these problems. In an attempt to explain what's happening, they

27

continue to blame others for their situation. If, for example, there's no longer joy in the bedroom, it must be that the wife is a shrew, not that alcohol is causing physical sexual inadequacy or that perhaps she's understandably not thrilled at being pawed by someone who's high on cocaine. As the negative consequences continue to mount, users suffer increasing distress, fear, and rejection, and often contemplate or attempt suicide. As they spend more and more time at the pain end of the continuum, the risk of suicide increases.

In interviewing several different groups of chemically dependent healthcare professionals now in recovery, it was found that 15% to 25% of the men and 23% to 38% of the women within each discipline had attempted suicide, some more than once. Many, many more had seriously considered it. These were obviously only the survivors, since the ones whose attempts succeeded were no longer available to answer questions, and we have no way of knowing accurately how many of them there were. The survivors said they had rarely left notes and had, on the contrary, gone to great lengths to make their attempts appear to be accidents so that children and other family would be spared as much pain as possible. Single-passenger automobile crashes and stepping out in front of trucks and buses were common methods, although drug overdose was the method of choice for both men and women. Many of the overdoses seem to have failed because there wasn't full awareness of how high the drug tolerance had become; amounts that should have proved lethal didn't.

4. Drinking/Using to Feel Normal

When chemical dependents can no longer achieve the desired effect from their drug and must drink or use just to move from pain to feeling normal, they've entered the final stage of the disease. The drug has lost its magical power to make them feel good or high; now it can bring them only to the original starting point. As an Anglican bishop once said, "The worst night was when I found that no matter how much I drank, I couldn't get drunk"—an echo of the psychologist who said, "After a while when I snorted I just had a nose caked with powder. I'd lost the high."

Without the drug, life is miserable, so they must have it, if only to relieve discomfort. But full relief from distress, conflict, and emotional pain is now very rare. Attempts to reduce these feelings lead to more accusations, self-deception, and blaming. Spouses, children, friends, co-workers, and employers are the most accessible targets. Active alcoholics and other drug users do estrange those who care the most about them. The lashing out at others, self-preoccupation, projection, and lack of emotional availability not only precipitate understandable hostility on the part of those around the chemically dependent person but compound the self-hatred and guilt of the one provoking the hostility. It's understandable how, when many professionals who haven't had timely intervention finally get to treatment, they've already alienated most of the significant persons in their lives. Husbands and wives who have stayed on in the situation often are frank to say their staying on didn't by then feel like loyalty or affection but only numbness and a kind of fatalistic acceptance.

This final stage of chemical dependence is just that, final. There's no turning back. There are truly only two alternatives at this point: either find a way to stop using alcohol/other drugs altogether, or face a major disaster such as loss of job and/or of license, or, in terms of physical disaster, brain damage or premature death.

Since reaching spontaneously for help is unlikely, prompt intervention by those who still care and are capable of action is the only reasonable alternative. As one woman religious put it in describing the members of her community, "They meant well, but they nearly loved and protected me to death."

Emotional Continuum, Stage 4

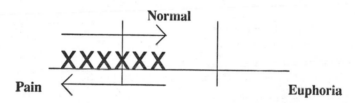

One hopes that as the various professions become more sophisticated in their knowledge of chemical dependence, they'll recognize the disease in their members long before the profound deteriorations characteristic of Stages 3 and 4 have set in—and will take prompt, helpful action.

Indicators of Chemical Dependence in the Professional

With each stage of chemical dependence **from Stage 2 on**, certain observable behaviors and changes accompany the increasing alcohol/other drug use. To categorize these symptoms, we've divided them below into three stages that correlate with the emotional syndrome just discussed.

An impaired professional may not exhibit all symptoms in any given stage, or may experience them in a different order. However, if several of them are obviously present, the others are usually there also. Single indicators are rarely diagnostic for chemical dependence; all indicators should be considered in a total assessment of the person's situation prior to intervention.

Stage 2: Seeking the Mood Swing

Indicators in Family/Social Systems
Gradual social withdrawal
Changes in family interaction
Behavioral changes (any deviations from normal personal or professional behavior)
Occasional intoxication
Frequent mood swings
Unpredictability
Isolation from friends
Poor stress tolerance
Dropping old companions in favor of drinking/using acquaintances

Indicators in All Professions
Suspicion of intoxication (alcohol/other drug use)
Unpredictability
Isolated incidents of questionable judgment or practice
Episodes of "forgetfulness"
Changes in office or hospital schedule
Withdrawal from professional committees or organizations
Defensiveness if questioned or confronted
Irritability
Adequate performance of required tasks, but unavailability for "extras"
Less creativity; coasting on reputation from previous work

Stage 3: Harmful Dependence

Indicators in Family/Social Systems
Lack of financial responsibility
Impulsive spending
Erratic behavior
Emotional withdrawal
Poor communication
DUI/DWI arrests/charges

Sexual dysfunction
Blackouts
Verbal, physical, or sexual abuse of spouse, children, friends, employees
Broken promises
Decline in health status: trauma, medical problems
Unkempt appearance at times
Episodes of public intoxication
Argumentativeness
Explosive outbursts of temper
Defensiveness or suspiciousness
Children often in trouble
Spouse less involved in activities outside the home

Indicators in All Professions
Erratic behavior
Observed poor judgment
Decline in quality of work
Client, patient, or other complaints
Nursing or office staff complaints
Changes in practice observed by colleagues
Frequent disruption of office or hospital schedule
Absences with elaborate explanations offered
Increased ordering of office-stock narcotics (in healthcare settings)
Questionable pharmacy practices (in healthcare settings)
Personal or professional behavior changes observed by office staff
Conflicts with colleagues or staff
Verbal abuse of office or hospital staff
Inappropriate behavior
Alcohol on breath, and attempts to cover with mints, mouthwash
Observed occurrences of intoxication, drowsiness, hypersensitivity during work hours
Deadlines barely met or missed altogether

Stage 4: Using to Feel Normal

Indicators in Family/Social Systems
Marked alienation from friends
Neglect of or giving up of social life, hobbies, or sports
Alienation from church, community groups
Marked family deterioration
Divorce or separation

Physical abuse of spouse, children
Increasing sexual dysfunction (impotence, frigidity, loss of desire)
Financial crisis
DUI/DWI or other legal action
Suicide attempts, often masked as accidents

Medical Symptoms
Observable decline in physical health
Weight changes
Pupils either dilated or constricted; face flushed/bloated (drinkers)
Serious medical illness
Emergency-room treatments: overdose, cellulitis, gastrointestinal prob-
lems, systemic infections, heart problems, burns, auto accidents, claims of
having been "mugged" but no witnesses

Indicators in Healthcare Professions
Gross malpractice
Errors in medication prescriptions
Unavailability when on call
Poor documentation of patient records
Questionable documentation on pharmacy records
Increased narcotic orders
Diversion from hospital, pharmacy, or office
Subject of medical staff review, possible disciplinary action

Indicators in the Legal Profession
Frequent failure to file required legal notifications
Missed deadlines
Failure to appear in court
Borrowing from or commingling of clients' trust funds
Slowness in processing mail, paying state bar dues

Indicators in All Professions
Obvious intoxication
Poor technical skills, tremors, blackouts, inability to concentrate
Staggering gait, disorientation, nodding off
Inappropriate behaviors
Unpredictable office, hospital, operating-room, church, or court schedule
Client or patient complaints
Clerical staff asked to make excuses or cover up for absences, uncompleted work

Chapter Highlights

Please note: These Chapter Highlights, to be found at the end of each chapter, are not to be taken as chapter **summaries** that repeat every main point made in a given chapter. In a book of this nature, many topics require quite lengthy and often complex treatment. As a result, any attempt at a brief summary of such topics would run the risk of oversimplification. So our policy has been to highlight only those points that can be rather easily repeated in brief form without distortion. For those who wish to review the main topics of a chapter quickly, the Contents pages will give that overview. For those who wish to review a chapter in more detail, scanning the main heads and numerous additional subheads in the text itself will give a much fuller picture of its contents.

Here are the highlights of Chapter 1:

The actual incidence of chemical dependence in the helping professions is difficult to document because:
- Many impaired professionals aren't reported to the licensing or certification boards.
- Many are simply fired from jobs and move on to other agencies, areas, or states.
- Cases reported to licensing boards haven't been specifically categorized as due to chemical dependence.
- Denial and concealment are common on the part of chemical dependents, their nuclear and extended families (friends, professional colleagues, and others). This is reflected in inaccurate death certificates and hospital discharge diagnoses.

Although we know that a significant number of our colleagues are affected by chemical dependence, we have difficulty identifying them because:
- We resist acknowledging to ourselves what we're seeing.
- We lack training in recognizing a chemically dependent person.
- We're reluctant to "accuse" a colleague without "proof."
- We just don't like to "get involved."

Chemical dependence is a primary, progressive, and fatal disease that can be treated. The disease is said to be present when there is:
- Loss of control over use of alcohol/other drugs
- Compulsive use of alcohol/other drugs
- Continued use of alcohol/other drugs in spite of the adverse consequences to the individual or to others

The emotional syndrome of chemical dependence as described by Vernon Johnson consists of four progressive stages of chemical use:
- Learning the mood swing
- Seeking the mood swing
- Harmful dependence
- Drinking or using to feel normal

The psychological dynamics of each of these stages effectively construct a wall of denial and delusion around the chemically dependent person, and the denial and delusion put him or her out of touch with reality.

Chapter 2

Enabling: A Major Block to Intervention

Enablers of the Chemically Dependent Professional

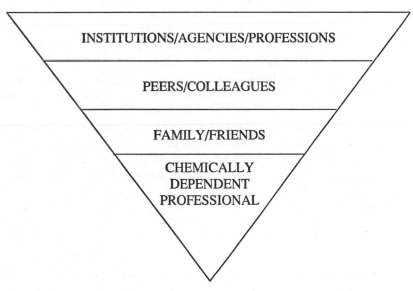

Enablers are people we'd all like to have as friends. They're usually ever-vigilant, loyal, caring, caretaking, and rescuing. They defend us to others, rationalize and excuse even our worst behavior, and try to help even when we haven't asked. These qualities, admirable in one sense, can be lethal in another. In the field of chemical dependence, "enabling" refers to those reactions or behaviors of family members, friends, or co-workers of chemical dependents that shield them from experiencing the harmful consequences of their alcohol/other drug use. Enablers encourage chemically dependent persons to continue their drinking or using by taking care of their responsibilities and assuming responsibility for their actions. Enablers are the most frequent roadblocks to intervention. Why and how this happens is complicated, but in this chapter we'll look at what families do and how we do much the same things in our professional roles.

How Families Enable

Secrets play an indispensable role in any society, including the family. But they have their dark side, too, as we'll see.

Family Secrets

For many of us, keeping secrets was a basic family rule, particularly if a family member was addicted to alcohol/other drugs. As kids we learned not to discuss family secrets with outsiders and sometimes not even with other members of the family. Many of us recall statements like "You shouldn't talk that way about your mother," "We don't want the neighbors to know our business," or "Anything that happens in this house stays in this house." We were also taught not to show others how we felt when something they did caused us pain or upset: "It's not ladylike to get angry," "Big boys don't cry," or "Put it out of your mind and it won't bother you." So we developed ways not only of keeping family secrets but also of detaching from or concealing our feelings. We learned that it's not acceptable to express feelings of hurt, anger, disappointment, or jealousy, so we became quite adept at hiding them or stuffing them. The principle that has come to pervade much of our society, then, is that to outsiders the family must maintain the image of stability and success; to all appearances this family **never** has a problem with anything. Of course, chemical dependence of a member is perceived as threatening the image of the perfect family. (As we'll point out, we naturally transfer those same family communication rules to our extended "family" of fellow professionals.)

So in a family where alcohol/other drugs create disturbances, members quickly mobilize to keep the dreaded secret. Despite the fact that chemical dependence has now achieved widespread visibility in this country and is at least intellectually accepted as a disease, many people still view it as social deviation or a moral weakness. The mental images of unkempt alcoholics lying in dark alleys or sipping from brown bags, or of other drug addicts stealing and mugging or stuporously wandering in the worst parts of the city looking for their next fix also serve to reinforce the idea that no such person is one of **our** family.

Enabling begins with denying the problem. We deny that our family member bears any resemblance to such people. In our constant attempts to maintain this defense, we minimize, cover up, and rationalize the effect that such members have on the family; we make excuses for their behavior and try to control their increasing alcohol/other drug use. We won't let this happen in our family. The enabling process is well underway.

Soon the "little white lie" becomes a habit. Perhaps it's a rationalization, a partial truth, or just a conscious omission of information, but all of these serve the same purpose of distorting the truth and misleading the inquisitive. Whether we even call this lying is determined for us by our colleagues, our parents, or other authority figures. If we were taught as children to say, "Dad couldn't come to the PTA meeting because he was sick," that was partially true. His speech was slurred, he slapped Mom and yelled at everyone else, and he did get sick later in the evening. Of course, the full truth is that he was intoxicated, but we were told to call it "sick," so this is exactly what we repeated at school. We were told, "Someone turned in front of Dad's car last night and caused an accident" when in fact Dad had been drinking and had run a red light. Over time, we learned a repertoire of excuses and explanations that substituted for the truth. A wife who's been beaten by her alcoholic husband explains to her employer that she slipped and hit her head on the corner of the coffee table. At the country club, a husband explains his drug-addicted wife's intoxicated behavior of last evening with "She didn't eat all day. That pain medication on an empty stomach really got to her."

Families all have secrets and myths. There are stories of infidelity, children born out of wedlock, sons who are gay, reasons why someone dropped out of school or left town that are never shared with the neighbors and usually not even with all the family. The habit of concealment may become pathological when alcohol/other drugs are involved. As loyal members of this family system we protect our own at all costs. And one huge cost to us is that we lose our ability to know what reality is—what the real truth is. Worse, we learn to devalue truth. And the cost to chemical dependents is that we hide the truth so well from ourselves and from outsiders that we won't permit the chemical dependents to be diagnosed as seriously ill. Simultaneously, our rationalizations, justifications, and rescuing effectively insulate them from the consequences of their alcohol/other drug use and rob them of the very experiences that might impel them toward recovery.

Nuclear Family Enabling Behaviors

Here are some of the commonest kinds of family enabling.

Making excuses and apologies to children for a chemically dependent adult's behavior or abuse: "Daddy wasn't feeling well; that's why he yelled at you." "Mom's upset lately; she just needs to relax and unwind. That's why she's drinking." "Dad had to work late again; that's why he couldn't come to your game." "No wonder your dad drinks every night, with all the noise you kids make."

Making excuses to employer for absences, tardiness, refusals to come to the phone, or for substandard work performance: "He's got the flu and feels lousy." "She's in bed with a migraine." "The car wouldn't start." "One of the kids is sick and I have to stay home." "Family emergency." "Death in the family." "Woke up with an awful toothache and had to spend the morning at the dentist's." Importantly, none of these illnesses is serious enough to warrant a medical clearance for returning to work. Most are presented as situations impossible to prevent or predict.

Helping the chemical dependent rationalize his or her use of alcohol/ other drugs and minimizing the effects: "You deserve to relax with a drink when you get home; you work too hard." "The doctor wouldn't have given you those pills to take unless you needed them." "Everyone gets a little high once in a while." "I guess you should have eaten before we went out." "I know things are pretty rough at work right now." "If he hadn't left it in the driveway you wouldn't have run over it." "The garage door isn't wide enough for that car anyhow."

Attempting to control the amount of the chemical dependent's use of alcohol/other drugs by manipulating the supply or the surroundings: Favorites are watering down the liquor, hiding extra liquor bottles that won't be missed, pouring weaker drinks, or telling a host to "go easy on his drinks," hiding drugs (particularly prescription drugs), getting rid of drugs found in the house. Other tricks are to get to a party late so that cocktail time is short, to take the alcoholic home early before there's too much drinking, and eventually to avoid altogether those times or places where alcohol/other drugs will be available.

Assuming responsibility for the chemical dependent's usual household tasks: Providing child care, cooking, shopping, paying bills, preparing taxes, taking care of household and car repairs, assuming responsibility for shopping, doing Christmas cards, and sending gifts and thank-you notes.

Attempting to reason with the chemically dependent person about alcohol/other drugs: "I really think you should cut down. It's not good for you." "Try to have just two drinks at the party. Last time you overdid it and got into a fight with Tom." "It's not good for the kids to see you drink so much."

Setting ultimatums and constantly backing down: "If you don't stop drinking, I'm leaving." "The next time you come home drunk I'm taking the children and not coming back." "The next time you're hung over and can't go to work I'm not making excuses for you." But nothing changes, and the threats are forgotten till next time.

Blaming the alcohol/other drug use on other circumstances and other people: "If they wouldn't push him so hard at work, he wouldn't drink so much." "If she didn't hang around with those people, she wouldn't use those drugs." "The other priests got him into it." "If we hadn't gotten a divorce the boy would never have started on drugs." "If her doctor didn't give her so many different prescriptions she wouldn't be like this, but I guess she needs them." "If he'd come straight home instead of going out with that bunch after work, he wouldn't drink so much." "He has to drink with colleagues. That's how the legislature works."

The habit of enabling becomes well entrenched with years of practice. As a result, chemical dependents rarely have to assume the consequences of their alcohol/other drug use. Comfortable and protected, they truly can't see reality because their families have distorted it so effectively for them and because they're investing much of their own psychic energy in denying it.

Professions as Family Systems

The helping professions, with their humanistic and caretaking missions, attract those who possess qualities of caring, giving, nurturing, perfectionism, and often genuine unselfishness and dedication. As neophytes we learn the expected behaviors of our professions—behaviors that reflect our commitment to those we serve—and we find that it really isn't too difficult to put our personal needs aside temporarily. Unfortunately, as this process continues we may gradually lose the balanced view of ourselves as whole people with a set of human needs and vulnerabilities like everyone else. Instead, we see ourselves more as helpers or fixers for everyone else.

In striving to meet the expectations of these helper or defender roles, we share with our colleagues a bond based on our common desire to contribute to the well-being of others. We now strongly align ourselves with those colleagues who profess the same ideals. We're inducted into a new "extended family" where we feel accepted, respected, and most importantly, needed. We're proud to be part of such an important enterprise. We share experiences and secrets unknown to laymen, things that might shock or frighten them if we even talk too freely. We work together, face uncertainty and pressure together, share a special kind of graveyard humor together, and help one another survive. An internship in any profession has much in common with a wartime foxhole experience; having been through either of them with others forges strong bonds. Only other clergy know what it's like to give spiritual solace day after day to the dying or to struggle to keep one's idealism in the face of a congregation that doesn't seem to want it. Only a fellow judge can know what it feels like to pass judgment on another human being and in the process wreck not only that person's life but that of a family watching helplessly as the criminal is led away.

So we need our professional families as we constantly practice our commitment to the family ideals by working long hours, working when we ourselves are ill, giving up our time off to fill in at work, and often placing our needs and those of our own families last in our priorities.

These behaviors are effectively reinforced by our colleagues and employers. "I don't know what we'd have done if you'd stayed out sick today." "Thanks for working the extra shift; you really bailed us out." The more this reinforcement happens, the more we accept our behavior as the norm. We develop the habit of responding first to others' needs and are rewarded by increased self-esteem. We must be doing the right things, since our colleagues, clients, and employers appreciate what we've done. We now truly identify ourselves as members of the professional family because our colleagues accept us—an acceptance symbolized by the process of licensure. We even possess legal documentation to prove that we belong.

How the Professions Enable

This professional family, much like our own nuclear families, is committed to maintaining an image for outsiders. The general public, namely those we serve, has traditionally viewed the helping professions as special. We have obligations imposed on us because we belong to this prestigious group: We must adhere to the practice statutes of licensure, conform to the image of our profession created by the public, and protect that image from harm. These expectations, though rather unrealistic, have placed the professions on the proverbial pedestal and thereby subject them to continuous public viewing and, in some cases, to increasing scrutiny and criticism. So when our profession is threatened by the public disclosure of some shameful event, we instinctively band together to protect our own, just as we do in our nuclear families. We hide from public view those things that we perceive as socially or morally unacceptable and detrimental to our positive image. We're deeply convinced, perhaps accurately so, that outsiders can't fully know or appreciate our professional lives and that only we should set and enforce standards for ourselves. Naturally, our goal is to keep unpleasant information a family secret. So unless we're ready to deal with the problem, certain facts must be hidden, distorted, explained away, or simply denied.

Organizational Enabling

While the nuclear family acts as a total system in the enabling process, it's comprised of one or more enablers. This also holds true for the helping professions. A total profession enables collectively through its organizations and institutions, but individual practitioners, supervisors, partners, and administrators enable **within** these organizations and institutions.

Many helping professions enable by their lack of knowledge about chemical dependence and by their unwillingness to learn or teach about it. When licensure or certification boards and bar associations complacently ignore chemical dependence and fail to devise systems to deal with members in a helpful, human way, they certainly can be classified as enablers. Most often, it's only when professionals' practice becomes severely affected by alcohol/other drug use that they end up before their respective bar associations, boards, or committees, and then only on disciplinary charges. Regulatory boards that don't address the issue of chemical dependence and simply punish the unacceptable behavior may discipline the individual professional but may never address its cause, that person's chemical dependence. Overreacting and doing so only very late, they lose the chance to motivate the person to go into treatment. For example, the diversion (stealing) of drugs from the hospital is a violation of the nursing practice act of any state, but if the board disciplines the nurse simply by suspending his or her license to practice, will that address the problem? Sick people don't get well just by being punished. Unfortunately, we know that despite the fact that the regulatory body of the profession has acted, this nurse's disease will continue to worsen whether he or she is licensed or not.

Unfortunately there are many such cases in all professions. One chemically dependent nurse had been diverting Demerol for about a year. The hospital finally identified the problem, fired her, reported her to the Board of Nursing, and referred her to a psychiatrist who placed her in an inpatient psychiatric setting for diagnosis. The psychiatrist determined that she wasn't addicted, since she showed no physical withdrawal symptoms. She was discharged but was to be seen on an outpatient basis by the psychiatrist. Her nursing license was suspended for one year. Since she had no skills other than familiarity with highly specialized nursing technology, she went to work at a veterinary clinic. While working there she was able to use on a small scale some of the same technical skills she had practiced for eight years.

One evening she found a box of narcotics in a back cupboard of the clinic. The dosages contained in the vials were ten times what would normally be found in a hospital, and there were ten vials! She took the vials, replaced the narcotics with Sodium Pentothal, an anesthetic, and began using them immediately. She wasn't discovered. She also admits to drinking during this period. Even though she didn't particularly enjoy alcohol, she felt it gave her some relief from her upset over what she had done and from her shame at losing her license.

After the year of suspension, she went before the board, promised she'd never steal drugs again, and regained her license to practice although she was to remain under probation for a year. While on probationary status she was required to communicate regularly with the board, submit progress reports from her employer, and have random urines screened for drugs by the local office of the Department of Regulation. She had a very difficult time finding employment in nursing because she had to admit to prospective employers why she was on probation. She did finally secure a night-shift position in an intensive care unit of a small hospital. After three months on the job she diverted drugs again and used "everything I could get my hands on" from the narcotic cabinet. She was escorted from the hospital in a stuporous condition and under arrest. The hospital notified the Board of Nursing, as it was obligated to do. The nurse was admitted to a second psychiatric hospital with a diagnosis of depression. Again, she was told she wasn't addicted—that the problem was her depression.

After her discharge from the hospital this nurse worked at a clerical job and was so severely depressed that she frequently wore the same clothes day after day. When her case was heard before the board she was so overwhelmed by hopelessness and shame that she voluntarily surrendered her license. Serendipitously, some eight months later she did get outpatient treatment for chemical dependence because of an accidental meeting with one of the authors. Two years after her arrest she pleaded her case before the board, documented her treatment and recovery through letters from counselors, physicians, and employers, and regained her nursing license. She's still being monitored but is drug-free and doing well.

The nursing board initially had no knowledge of how to deal with chemical dependence. Instead of offering real help, it simply resorted to disciplinary action because the nurse's behavior met the criteria for professional misconduct according to the professional practice act of the state (i.e., the state's rules and regulations for professional practice within its jurisdiction). The end result was that this nurse, like many others, was allowed to progress in her disease without intervention that would have specifically addressed it. The liability here was heavy indeed, since without chemical dependence treatment the nurse remained dangerous to herself and potentially dangerous to others even after her term of punishment had been completed and her license reinstated.

Institutional Enabling

Institutions such as agencies, hospitals, and universities that house our professional families also have very effective patterns of enabling. These institutions often enable by simply ignoring the problem of chemical dependence. If we admit that such a problem exists, we're obligated to develop policies that reflect an institutional philosophy and to spell out procedures to be followed when suspected chemical dependence surfaces. Without formal policies and procedures, these institutions and the persons within them are left to ignore the problem or to improvise. It's then not hard to understand how the physician can appear repeatedly with alcohol on his breath before appropriate measures are taken, or how the nurse can be suspected of diverting narcotics but allowed to continue because proof didn't force itself on her colleagues. Or the administrator may have a heavy odor of alcohol on his breath, slurred speech, and forgetfulness, but no one in the organization will inititate action. "It's not my job!" True, but that's because it's not yet anyone's job.

This institutional neglect isn't very different from that of the family system we talked about earlier, except that now we apply those family rules to our professional life. We keep our secrets, and above all we never needlessly rock the boat by voicing our concerns or suspicions—not when we ourselves are passengers in that boat and want it to sail smoothly.

When our professions deny chemical-dependence problems, they also accept, at least tacitly, enabling behavior. Unwittingly we fall into the trap of following the rules. And rules aren't new to us. We've already adapted to the expectations of our birth families and adopted the mores of a profession; now we've taken on yet another code of expected behaviors: that of the individual institution, agency, or organization in which we work and to which we belong. Men in particular, but women also, are praised for being team players and punished for moving against the crowd.

Here is a list of some specific enabling behaviors common to institutions and to persons within them. Note that most of these behaviors can be traced to two broad failings: 1) lack of policies and procedures that define chemical dependence in employees and that lay down specific ways to deal with it, and 2) lack of education about what chemical dependence is, how certain attitudes affect our ability to deal with the problem, and how chemical dependence affects persons in the workplace. But to specifics:

1. Lack of training programs for management-level personnel regarding identification, documentation, and how to intervene with chemically dependent employees
2. Lack of employee assistance programs to assist with identification, treatment, and referrals for chemical dependence
3. Lack of competency-oriented job-performance evaluations; poor documentation of that performance, especially of events or behaviors that may indicate chemical dependence
4. Lack of defined absenteeism and tardiness policies related to the use of alcohol/other drugs
5. Reluctance to cooperate with licensing boards or bar associations to collect data about a chemically dependent professional
6. Inconsistent disciplinary responses to suspected intoxication on duty
7. Reinforcing "keeping the secret" rules by rationalizing or minimizing specific behaviors exhibited by a professional or other staff member suspected of chemical dependence
8. Lack of employee insurance benefits to cover treatment of chemical dependence
9. Unfamiliarity with available resources and procedures to be following in making reports on or obtaining help for a suspected chemically dependent employee

One of the more dramatic examples of institutional enabling we know concerned a small community hospital where the nurse who did intravenous therapy was suspected of diverting drugs. Numerous staff reports had been filed with the Director of Nursing regarding her asking for the narcotic keys when she was on a patient unit. She was also frequently seen looking through patients' medication records. Since as an I.V. nurse she had no responsibility for administering any controlled drugs or oral pain medications, her behavior was suspicious. The hospital's solution to her problem was to change a policy so that only one nurse controlled the keys on each shift. All the keys were changed as well. Nothing else was done.

Enabling by Work Groups

Now we move into the most direct and immediate area of enabling: that done by work groups (which of course often includes many colleagues and friends). The work group will vary from perhaps two to three people for a dentist or veterinarian in private practice to over a hundred for a busy faculty member, counselor, partner in a major law firm, or hospital physician. In all these groups the individuals function along much the same lines as do members of the family systems we've talked about. Here we're talking about the set of rules established by the work group.

This group is at the heart of our daily activities, and our role within it reinforces our identity as a helper, caretaker, professional. On a deeper level, we're of course meeting our need to be loved, to belong, to be accepted. Our mere presence in this group does this for us day after day. We care about and for each other, rescue each other, comfort each other and, yes, enable each other. Of course we don't consciously make a choice to hide signs and symptoms of chemical dependence or of any other major problem, for that matter. Rather we see ourselves as helping in some way. These helping behaviors may be as subtle as repeating explanations and filling in for co-workers when they're late or absent, accepting their mistakes when they're preoccupied, forgetful, angry, disorganized, or depressed. Often we share their personal problems and concerns and find it easy to understand why they're acting the way they are. Most of them have done similar favors for us over the years, and we've appreciated their acceptance and help when we weren't at our best. So we dismiss their unusual or inappropriate behavior as simply responses to a temporary crisis or problem at home. This is easy to do when the chemically dependent person tells us he or she is having personal problems or doesn't feel well. Of course, what we may miss is that the progressive behavioral changes often causing these problems are a direct result of increasing alcohol/other drug use.

To complicate matters further, our colleague may also complain of physical problems that may warrant medical treatment or hospitalization. This real and documented illness may provide another cause for our rationalizing the performance problems we've observed. The illness also sometimes creates an opportunity for chemically dependent persons to obtain drugs legitimately, and this enhances their own denial of any inappropriate use. Dealing with medically ill chemically dependent professionals can be a challenge. When hospitalized they may receive increased doses of pain medication, since they may already have developed tolerance to particular drugs or may even begin to exhibit withdrawal symptoms. Without assessment by knowledgeable medical or nursing staff, this may progress into a dangerous withdrawal situation without anyone's anticipating or recognizing the problem.

If the chemical dependence is identified while the professional is hospitalized, what then? The physician in charge of the case should then address the problem. However, if the patient is in healthcare, the physician is a member of the same enabling family. In that case, even if the situation is correctly diagnosed and the suspected alcohol/other drug use mentioned, the discussion will usually go no further. Unfortunately, the episode will often falsely reassure friends and co-workers that they were wrong in their suspicions, since they believe that in the course of diagnosis for another illness, any addiction problems would of course be discovered and treated. This false reassurance will lead to more delay and rationalization.

It's common for a friend or spouse to urge a trip to a personal physician for a good checkup in hopes that the physician will see the alcohol/other drug problem and take things in hand. But since the physician knows nothing about what's going on at home or office and since the patient comes for a routine physical, the addiction will almost certainly be missed unless there's some very obvious physical sign. If, as is usually the case, the physician has received little or no formal training in how to recognize or manage chemical dependence, very little of benefit will occur. The patient won't volunteer much information, and the physician probably won't suspect the problem or ask about it.

In hospitals it's not uncommon for physicians to quickly write a prescription for a nurse or other hospital staff member in the hallway or on a nursing unit. The medication may be a pain reliever, muscle relaxant, tranquilizer, or other drug that the staff member says is needed to alleviate a temporary problem. It's important here to remember: 1) The physician is responding to a "family member" who's asking for help now so he or she can continue working, and 2) healthcare professionals know that medications do solve many problems. This is enabling at its finest. The physician is responding as caretaker and acts in the belief that this is a helping gesture. What the physician may not know is that the person ostensibly being helped is chemically dependent and is also obtaining prescriptions from other physicians, none of whom thinks of comparing notes or keeping records.

Many of us, then, are enablers on one level or another, for one person or another, not necessarily only to the chemically dependent. We enable our colleagues, friends, family members, and even our clients and patients, though usually with no serious consequences. But when we enable chemically dependent persons, especially where a pattern of frequent use of increasing amounts of alcohol/other drugs has developed, we're enabling a very dangerous problem to continue and worsen.

A nurse who was a long-term employee in a hospital had been developing unusual behavior patterns. His patient care, which had always been very thorough and of excellent quality, had become haphazard, and he often did just enough to get by. He was seen covering a patient's soiled bed with Chux rather than changing it, leaving patients to wait long periods for pain medication, being abrupt with patients, and handling them roughly. These problems were noted mostly by the shift following his and were reported rather sporadically to the head nurse. Colleagues on his own shift noted a change in how he related to them. Formerly outgoing, cheerful, and talkative, over a period of several months he became withdrawn and isolated. They attributed this change to known difficulties in his marriage. In fact, the staff attributed most of the changes in his behavior and patient care to these personal problems.

Other staff members followed behind him almost routinely, fixed his omissions in patient care, changed empty intravenous bottles for him, cleaned his patients who had remained in soiled beds, and took notes for him at staff meetings when he was increasingly late to work—all in an attempt to be helpful. Over the years he had developed close relationships with his colleagues, and he was well liked. Later it was difficult to obtain actual data from them regarding the deterioration of his professional performance.

Interestingly, the attempt to get him some help was finally precipitated by a co-worker who observed him placing small plastic bags from the pharmacy into his knapsack; meanwhile, another co-worker reported to the charge nurse that one of his patients was crying in pain. The chart indicated that the patient had been medicated two hours before, but the patient, who was alert and oriented, said she had received nothing for her pain. The co-worker couldn't see if there were any medications in the pharmacy bags (the bags that contain patient medications sent from the pharmacy with a label stating the patient's name, medication, and dosage amount for a twenty-four-hour period). But the co-worker did question the nurse and was told the bags were empty and that he was taking them home to use as containers for nails and screws in his workshop. However, he didn't offer to demonstrate that this was true.

On that same shift, several other omissions in patient care were brought to the attention of the charge nurse. The charge nurse discussed the situation with the head nurse and Director of Nursing, who then notified the peer assistance program. The program sent an advocate—a professional trained in identifying and intervening with chemically dependent professionals. When the advocate met with the Director of Nursing, the head nurse, and the assistant head nurse, he was told that the nurse needed help only because he was having "some personal problems."

It was evident from this meeting that chemical dependence was still the last thing on their minds. In fact, they reacted defensively to the advocate's suggestion that the behavioral changes, mood swings, negligence in patient care, and the pharmacy bags in the nurse's knapsack strongly suggested an alcohol/other drug problem. The Director of Nursing clearly stated, "I know it's not that kind of problem." While exploring other behavioral documentation with this group, the advocate asked to review the narcotic records and random patient charts. The discrepancies between what was signed out on the narcotic records and documented in the patient charts were minimal, but there were several occasions where a narcotic was signed out and not recorded on a patient chart, and one instance of several doses signed out for the same patient in much too short a time. The assistant head nurse, when asked about any unusual occurrences related to patient medications, did say that their shift frequently had to reorder certain patient medications. (At this hospital the pharmacy sends a 24-hour supply of ordered patient medications to the unit, which means there should be no need to special-order a medication from the pharmacy.)

The peer assistance advocate next asked about any known physical changes. Both the head nurse and the assistant head nurse had noted that the nurse, who used to be meticulous about his appearance, had frequently been unshaven, had worn wrinkled uniforms, and had lost a significant amount of weight. He frequently looked tired and strained and had dark circles under his eyes. Neither the assistant head nurse nor the head nurse had consciously put together the picture that was taking shape. With each additional piece of information they appeared more distressed, not only because they had been blind to obvious signs of chemical dependence but also because of the implications of the new interpretation. They were genuinely fond of this man and didn't want to find that he was chemically dependent.

After consultation with other hospital authorities an intervention took place, evaluation with a local addiction specialist was scheduled immediately, and a bed secured for admission at a local chemical dependence treatment center. The nurse agreed to the recommendation that he go to residential treatment and also agreed to give a urine specimen immediately after the intervention. When he was admitted that day he brought with him in his knapsack all the small plastic pharmacy bags with their medication labels. He admitted to taking the whole array of drugs: tranquilizers, antibiotics, antidepressants, and others—in addition to drinking heavily.

Even after intervention the supervisory nursing team of Director of

Nursing, assistant head nurse, and head nurse still had difficulty accepting the reality of the chemical dependence problem. Small wonder that they had failed to identify the situation earlier! They were the enablers, as were the many other staff who had so kindly and caringly tried to help by completing the nurse's assignments and doing for him the things he had neglected. None of them consciously made a choice to ignore the truth, but their personal involvement with the nurse made them unable to view his behavior and performance objectively. They had innocently delayed the identification of the chemical dependence through rescuing, denial, rationalizing, and excusing.

We enable our chemically dependent colleagues by covering up when they're late, absent, preoccupied, forgetful, angry, disorganized, depressed. We make excuses, right their mistakes, apologize for their rudeness, and cover their tracks. We do all of this because we care. Like the supervisor who allowed a physician assistant to sleep off an overdose in a patient's room, we want to protect our colleagues, not harm them. But in the process we're burying the data that might lead to early and helpful intervention. Each time we correct a mistake, excuse an obvious bit of misbehavior, conceal an apparent shortage while making out a drug count report, or fill in for a colleague in court, we hide the truth. When a formerly reliable person isn't performing up to standard, there's something wrong! After all, reasonable, conscientious people don't deliberately choose to become irresponsible.

During the data collection process you'll repeatedly see enabling much as we've described it. Workers know something is wrong, but they're reluctant to document anything for fear of facing a colleague's anger or retaliation, fear that harm will come to a friend because of what they disclose, fear that they'll lose their own places as loved and trusted members of the group if they seem to be disloyal. Taught from childhood that no one likes a tattletale, and well aware of their own imperfections, they hesitate to finger someone else lest the same thing happen to them.

Administrative personnel are also plagued with denial and enabling. While they may have been aware of a problem for some time and even discussed it with an individual, the problem is often called something else— but it stubbornly persists. In fact, administrators and executives often say flatly, "We don't have that problem here"—denial that not only absolves them from the stigma of having chemically dependent staff, colleagues, friends, or family members but allows them to continue or even step up their enabling.

Anyone working as an intervenor will certainly find enablers. Chemical dependents can't long survive and continue to drink and use without them. They'll of course challenge would-be intervenors but should never surprise them. If intervenors are key persons they must be educated about chemical dependence as a disease and about what it costs if it's allowed to progress—costs both personal and professional. This education must be given if we're going to gain their confidence and enlist their aid in the data collection process. Be patient. They may vacillate about the need for intervention and look for easier, less demanding alternatives. If so, you must constantly reassure them and keep restating the facts.

The husband of a pharmacist called the peer assistance program for help for his wife who "was stealing drugs from the hospital." He had found a bag full of drugs in a cabinet in the house and knew she had taken them from the hospital. He suspected she was using drugs because she had been acting strangely and was defensive and evasive when he questioned her. He brought the bag full of drugs to a meeting with the peer assistance team and the Director of Pharmacy. The plastic bag contained syringes and a large amount of oral medications, sedatives, tranquilizers, synthetic opiates, all with the hospital pharmacy sticker on them. Even when told of this evidence, the Director of Pharmacy denied that it could be true. He insisted the pharmacist was excellent and had no work-related problems. Despite the husband's observations, the Director found it impossible to believe that this pharmacist could possibly be taking drugs. But when the husband brought in the bag of drugs and actually placed them on the director's desk, he finally had to accept the concrete evidence.

Am I an Enabler? A Self-Inventory

It has been our experience that at least 90% of professionals we have interacted with have worked with or known a colleague who was chemically dependent. For many, though, the enabling wasn't identified. While thinking about those you have known, answer yes or no to the following statements about possible enabling on your part.

Am I an Enabler? A Self-Inventory

1. I believe that the professionals I personally come in contact with are above having chemical dependence problems.

2. I fear for my own position if I were to take action on a colleague's chemical dependence problem.

3. I'm hesitant to confront a colleague about his or her alcohol/other drug use for fear of anger or rejection.

4. I've covered up a colleague's alcohol/other drug use.

5. I excuse colleagues' alcohol/drug-related behavior as atypical or as attributable to other problems.

6. I accept responsibility for my colleagues' duties, assignments, or caseload, even when I suspect that the reasons given for their failure to perform well aren't valid.

7. I become increasingly angry at my colleagues for not carrying their share of the workload.

8. I believe that chemical dependence is a sign of moral weakness.

9. I believe that any professional could stop drinking or using if he or she really wanted to.

10. I sometimes worry about my own patterns of alcohol/other drug use, but I mention this only to others who drink or use other drugs much as I do and who will reassure me.

11. I tend to avoid colleagues who might have a chemical dependence problem.

12. I'm fearful of what a superior might do if I express my concerns about a colleague's alcohol/other drug use.

13. I hesitate to tell a colleague directly how I feel about his or her behavior, especially when I suspect the behavior is alcohol/other drug-related.

14. I've defended and made excuses for a chemically dependent colleague.

15. I fear that if I identify colleagues' chemical dependence they may lose their licenses.

16. I've failed to act on complaints about a colleague's suspected alcohol/other drug use or have passed them along only to those who are unlikely to do anything about them.

17. I've ignored or denied suspicions about a potential chemical dependence problem in a colleague.

18. I've written prescriptions for a colleague who isn't my patient, or for myself, or for my own family.

19. I postpone action when I suspect that a colleague is chemically dependent; I trust time, other people, or changes in circumstance to solve the problem.

Chapter Highlights

Chemically dependent professionals don't exist in isolation. They're encouraged to keep using alcohol/other drugs by enabling families, professions, institutions, and colleagues. These enablers are major roadblocks to early intervention, and in their attempts to help the chemically dependent person they too distort reality. While the alcohol/other drug use is causing problems in our colleagues' family, social, spiritual, and professional lives, those who care the most about them are protecting them from experiencing the consequences of their use.

Family/friends enable by:
- making excuses for the chemical dependent's inappropriate behavior
- making excuses for tardiness, absenteeism, or lower-quality work
- rationalizing and minimizing the chemical dependent's use of alcohol/other drugs
- attempting to control the family member's alcohol/other drug use
- assuming responsibility for the chemical dependent's usual tasks
- rarely following through with ultimatums regarding the alcohol/other drug use
- blaming circumstances or others for the family member's alcohol/other drug use

Professional groups enable by:
- fostering unrealistic ideals and expectations of the professional
- remaining uneducated regarding the disease of chemical dependence
- promoting the keeping of "family secrets" by denying chemical dependence among colleagues
- disciplining their chemically dependent colleagues instead of assisting them to get help
- acting only when cases are far advanced and problems are very obvious

Institutions enable by:
- promoting the keeping of secrets about chemical dependence problems among staff to avoid upset, save face, and/or avoid litigation
- denying the need for educational programs about chemical dependence
- not having adequate employee insurance and other benefits that cover treatment of chemical dependence
- failing to develop written policies and peer assistance programs

Colleagues enable by:
- believing that chemical dependence can't happen to a professional
- making excuses for a chemically dependent colleague's behavior or performance
- minimizing the obvious effects of alcohol/other drug use in a friend or colleague
- rationalizing changes in a chemically dependent colleague's performance, behavior, or appearance
- covering up for a chemically dependent colleague's errors or omissions
- writing prescriptions for a chemically dependent colleague without complete medical assessment or without recording the action in the colleague's medical chart

Chapter 3

The Solution: Intervention

A chemically dependent professional is always someone else's problem. Unfortunately, the someone else often doesn't know what to do about it. One surgeon repeatedly showed up to operate with the odor of alcohol on his breath. He looked rather disheveled until he had changed into his greens and headgear. At times his hands seemed shaky. This went on for months. The nursing staff reported it to the nursing supervisor, who in turn reported it to the Director of Nursing, who reported it to the Chief of Medical Staff, who said he'd talk to the surgeon. Perhaps he did, but nothing changed. The problem continued.

Finally one night the surgeon appeared in the emergency room grossly intoxicated, and a patient's complaint to the hospital administration finally got results. The nurses involved in this incident had tried to help but didn't know what to do when appeal to a higher authority failed. The surgeon ultimately was successfully referred to treatment, not through intervention at the first clear signs of trouble, but only much later and as an alternative to inevitable disciplinary action by the Medical Board. While the hospital staff did nothing, patients were undoubtedly in jeopardy.

A major misconception among professionals is that they must be able to **prove** that someone is using alcohol/other drugs while on duty. It's unclear why that notion persists in the face of obvious substandard practice, which deserves challenge whatever its cause. Still, even in spite of symptoms that intrude on the workplace, supervisors and colleagues feel immobilized until they have absolute proof. Also there's a gray area when the drug is alcohol. Most social functions include alcohol. It's an accepted, sometimes even encouraged, part of celebrating and unwinding, and a reward after a hard day's work. Just as attorneys share a few drinks as part of a working lunch or a group of priests may drink together before dinner, healthcare professionals, nurses in particular, are known to go out for a drink together after work. Hospital policies on drinking may be vague or nonexistent, so Christmas parties are held on the premises, and staff may drop in to share a drink or two before going to the floors to finish rounds. One physician, head of an obstetrics-gynecology department, regularly enjoyed cocktails at lunch before seeing outpatients in the afternoon but didn't understand why his house staff then assumed it was all right to drink at dinner before nights on call.

So who feels entirely secure in whistle blowing because someone drinks before work or comes in smelling of alcohol? Most people drink, and professionals are rarely off duty. One drink or several smell much the same. When there's an emergency, professionals respond, regardless of what they've been doing. Short of total abstinence at all times except on vacations, how can professionals always manage never to work after some drinking? Most professions do have principles that define the use of alcohol during work hours as unprofessional and even as grounds for disciplinary action, although few hospitals or social agencies or institutions have written policies that forbid any work at all after drinking or that specify how much time must pass. One obvious exception is the airline industry, which has stringent rules and regulations governing the use of alcohol/other drugs by pilots and flight attendants during and before work hours. The reason is clear: The safety of passengers and cargo is critical. But are patients or clients of alcohol/other drug-impaired physicians or lawyers in any less danger?

When we speak of the chemically dependent person, we're talking about a very serious matter. Frequent or consistent odor of alcohol on the breath during work hours (or the telltale smell of breath mints to mask it) can be a very late-stage symptom, predictably preceded by other changes as well. The director of a hospital-based employee assistance program says, "An alcoholic nurse or doctor is like a germ in a petri dish. Trouble grows and spreads."

If we look beyond the alcohol/other drug use, we can usually identify practice-related clues that provide objective, indisputable data for intervention. For example, the surgeon we just mentioned was repeatedly late for his cases and held up the operating-room schedule. While operating he took longer than necessary with basic general surgery procedures. At times he totally forgot to write the patient's post-op orders and made several errors in writing medication orders as well. This information alone should have initiated the intervention even without information from the staff regarding his obvious intoxication and mood swings. Reporting the use of alcohol is really secondary in preparing data for the intervention, even though its role in causing the problems is primary. Once understood, this removes some of the gray area. One is spared seeming to sit in judgment on colleagues, lecturing them about drinking that they may argue differs only to a minor degree, if that, from what others do. Professionals have less difficulty in defining acceptable standards of practice, particularly in their own field, so they're the ones most able to collect and evaluate data for intervention.

The Basics of Intervention

Intervention, as defined by Vernon Johnson, the "father of intervention," means presenting reality in a receivable way to a person who's out of touch with it. The goal of intervention is simply to get the chemically dependent person to accept help (treatment). It certainly doesn't sound difficult, but remember that we're attempting to get help accepted by people who think it's the last thing they need. For doing this, the Johnson Institute intervention model has proven ideal in most situations, particularly those involving family members. However, in preparing to intervene with professional colleagues we have to adapt the model somewhat to allow for a different approach, as we'll see.

Why Interventions with Colleagues Are Different

Although some professional peer assistance programs do include families in interventions with professionals, most often these interventions with professionals involve only colleagues. In any setting, intervention is based on the information, observations, and concerns of significant persons regarding the chemically dependent person. When **colleagues** are reporting the information and concerns, though, what they're able to present is quite different, and the power they hold is different.

There are other reasons why we usually don't include families. One issue of concern is the chemically dependent professional's right to confidentiality. If colleagues identify problems related to practice or job performance, they don't necessarily have the right to share that information with the colleague's family. So their obligation is to act on the information and yet ensure confidentiality to the greatest degree possible. There's also a real risk that a family member alerted to the coming intervention will in turn alert the person who needs the intervention, bring in lawyers, and lose the element of surprise that would help the intervention succeed. Most families, as we mentioned earlier, have become deeply involved in enabling behaviors, and so they often react protectively or defensively without waiting to learn what the intervention is about or what's being planned.

Significant others who aren't professional colleagues are sometimes a primary source of referrals to treatment programs and may sometimes contribute data about a person's social and private life. Sometimes family members or significant others do participate in interventions from the very beginning when they've served as the initial whistle-blowers, but interventions by colleagues in the workplace more often than not are done without their participation. A spouse invited to participate may well sabotage the entire project, since family members may be even more adamant than the chemical dependent in denying the problem and may even be deeply involved with alcohol/other drugs themselves and far from eager to make changes. If they're to be included, avoid problems by carefully evaluating in advance their ability to participate.

Who and How Many Should Do An Intervention?

Interventions with colleagues involve two or more significant persons (usually professional colleagues) who have exact, specific, documented information about someone's social, personal, and professional behaviors related to alcohol/other drug use that have created concern. Intervenors may be professional partners, friends, colleagues, or a combination of people in positions of authority, such as a hospital administrator, a representative of a program for the impaired, a person who's now in recovery, a professional intervention expert, or someone else. There's no simple formula for how many people to involve except to say that one should never attempt intervention **alone**. Because chemical dependence is characterized by denial and the affected person is often severely deluded, solo attempts are usually disastrous.

Teams of at least two persons are recommended for the purposes of maintaining objectivity and for helping each other withstand attempts the subject will almost certainly make to attack, project, blame, and rationalize. Because there may be differences in how the event is remembered and reported, it helps to have at least one other person who can attest to what really took place and what was agreed to. Furthermore, a team of (at least) two works very effectively with persons in advanced stages of chemical dependence because the situation quite naturally demands that two rather different messages be delivered: the hard "bottom line" message of what will happen if the impaired professional doesn't comply with the team's request that he or she get an evaluation, and the equally necessary message of empathy and loving concern. One team member in effect becomes the "bad guy" who delivers the harsh news, and the other becomes the "good guy" who tells the subject just as sincerely and nonthreateningly something like "The information we gathered from many people shows that you really have a problem. Your friends and co-workers are very concerned about you and want you to have help. That's why we're here." The twofold message usually works very well.

Another very practical reason for having at least two people on the team is physical safety: both the subject's and your own. Paranoia is common in chemical dependents and may appear unexpectedly, both because of the physiological effects of the drug and because of what has probably been progressive personal disruption (loss of family, friends, financial security, for example) and the new impending threat to career and status that intervenors represent. People who feel under attack can become violent or suicidal and act out their angry feelings. On rare occasions a chair, telephone, or book has been known to hit the wall. One intervention led to a chipped ankle when a seemingly meek clergyman became enraged and threw a phone receiver; unfortunately, a church elder's ankle was in the line of fire. Although these incidents are extremely rare, it's best to be forewarned. (We'll discuss safety further when explaining preparation for intervention.) A safe rule is to include as many people as necessary without overwhelming the chemically dependent professional.

What Is the Basis for Intervention?

The **what** (or what for) of intervention is the heart of the matter. What requires action now? What used to be different, and what's gone wrong? In other words, what brought the problem to light? What are the specific professional practice issues? What are the observable and documentable behavioral changes? What changes have staff noticed in the way the person attends to work schedules, client or patient interactions, staff interactions, and other professional obligations? These questions should be answered with concrete, specific examples, not generalizations. Usually one precipitating event sets the wheels in motion, but there's usually also a progression of many events that can be recalled later. Each might be explained away easily if taken in isolation, but the cumulative effect of single episodes presented one after another can, like the threads that the Lilliputians used to bind Gulliver, be very powerful. Unacceptable behavior related to specific events and incidents must be documented as completely as possible, and client and patient records must be reviewed, as well as narcotic records if pertinent.

A 28-year-old male nurse working in a cardiac intensive care unit was seen to develop increasingly marked personality changes. Other staff attributed them to the death of his father six months earlier. He was increasingly emotionally unpredictable and at times explosive. Also other staff had complained to the head nurse that he insisted on taking Bed #1 every day. (This was a bed always assigned to a fresh post-operative open-heart patient.) Other staff found this irritating, since the care of the Bed # 1 patient was stimulating and fast-paced, and they enjoyed this type of nursing challenge. Eventually the staff noticed that he no longer would go to lunch with them. He was frequently leaving the unit, and they had received several complaints from patients' families about his uncaring attitude. This behavior was very unlike this man, so co-workers began questioning what was wrong with him.

A new head nurse was assigned to the unit, and she soon identified the nurse as probably in trouble with drugs. The narcotics records, in addition to the other symptoms, painted a very clear picture.The Bed #1 nurse was usually assigned responsibility for the narcotic count. Still, there never appeared to be any narcotics missing. He had been forging patients' names and other nurses' names and ordering a full box at a time. At the time of discovery he was using 800 mg of Demerol at a single injection and had been diverting drugs for over a year, but he wasn't identified until an outsider, the new head nurse, came to this unit. The other staff had chosen to rationalize and excuse the nurse's performance as grief-related rather than looking at an obvious problem of drug use.

When to Intervene

Frequently professionals have difficulty deciding when to intervene. How much data is actually needed to proceed with an intervention? How serious do things need to be? Simply, if you're suspicious and see the symptoms listed in Chapter 1, under Indicators of Chemical Dependence in the Professional, the illness is probably well along and intervention is indicated. Remember, by the time there's observable deterioration in professional practice, there's probably significant deterioration in other areas of the person's life outside of work that he or she is finding increasingly difficult to hide. This is the time to intervene if you think the problem is alcohol/other drug use. Colleagues tend to be under-suspicious rather than over-suspicious. We can cite many situations where serious alcohol/other drug-related problems have been ignored, misread, or denied, but we rarely encounter a situation where suspecting chemical dependence has occurred too early or with no justification. Even then, it wasn't that there was no problem or that intervention wasn't needed. The problem was that alcohol/other drugs and severe mental illness were intertwined in ways that cast the emphasis wrongly on the chemical dependence.

All too often colleagues avoid a planned formal intervention even in situations where a problem is obvious. They attempt to diagnose the problem themselves by deciding to refer to psychiatrists, marital counselors, employee assistance programs, or spiritual counselors, depending on their own perceptions of the case. These referrals, for a chemical dependent who is in denial and is severely deluded, are generally ineffective for several reasons. A therapist working on a one-to-one basis is often not aware of the full situation, deals only with the identified patient, and never learns the whole story, a story that the patient can't or won't tell. The patient will "con" the therapist by focusing on other personal problems—such as marriage problems, child problems, medical problems—as reasons for the referral, minimizing or denying the alcohol/other drug use. These patients may terminate any counseling relationship shortly after its initiation by rationalizing "I can't afford it," "I did get help and I'm better now," or "I've been trying, but it's not helping. Nothing is any better."

Also, when a confidential relationship exists between counselor and counselee, the counselor usually can't obtain needed information about the client's current situation without permission. So it's easy to see how therapists are duped by people frightened that their alcohol/other drug use will become known. Probably the greatest disadvantage of this referral approach is that it allows the illness to continue and delays more definitive treatment. It gives the illusion that the problem is being solved when often it's unchanged or worsening.

Yet there are ways to avoid the double trap of either overlooking serious psychiatric illness by assuming that everything is attributable to alcohol/other drugs or, at the other extreme, of referring the person to a mental-health professional who knows little or nothing about chemical dependence. Once the problem is understood, the solution appears obvious. The person will be sent for evaluation or admission at once to a treatment facility that specializes in alcohol/other drug dependence but that also has competent psychiatrists available so that evaluation for other possibilities is part of the initial assessment. If the person is sent to a therapist, that therapist must have expertise in evaluating chemical dependence, and the person being referred must agree that the intervenors may tell the therapist the full history that led to the referral and that the therapist will tell the referring person(s) exactly what the patient and therapist decide. There must also be agreement that communication between referrer and therapist will remain open. Otherwise there may be continued drinking/using, or the patient may simply stop seeing the therapist. Without a planned system for alerting the referrer that this is happening, the patient is free to use alcohol/other drugs as much as he or she wishes (or is clever enough to conceal) while colleagues and employers innocently believe the situation has been handled.

A 30-year-old nurse working the evening shift was described by her director as exhibiting "symptoms of stress." Her moods were up and down, she was hostile toward co-workers, made numerous medication errors, and provoked complaints from patients. When she called in sick and her speech seemed slurred, it was explained as extreme fatigue. There had also been frequent discrepancies in the narcotic signout book on this unit, but the director didn't see them as related. The nurse had moved from another state and seemingly had no local support system, so the nursing department referred her to a psychiatrist to help her work through her difficulties. She enrolled in weekly counseling and was prescribed anti-depressants. Her performance didn't improve. The nurse claimed that the medication was making her tired all the time. Her practice worsened, and the director called the peer assistance program. After her history and records were examined, an intervention was scheduled. The psychiatrist was contacted, and although she could not divulge information, the background for the intervention was explained to her. The nurse was then admitted to an inpatient chemical dependence hospital treatment center for evaluation. It was determined that she had been diverting and using Demerol for over six months and also using other drugs outside the hospital.

The **when** of this case was the point at which the director identified particular professional practice behaviors that weren't acceptable and didn't reach the level of performance expected of this particular nurse. The director was able to collect data to refer this nurse informally to counseling. Why didn't she intervene instead? The administration of this hospital was unfamiliar with the indicators of chemical dependence in the workplace and also didn't understand that the burden of proof was not on the hospital. The director chose a familiar path, a referral to a mental-health professional. Having done so and with the treatment process underway, she felt she had met her obligation and had no need to dig deeper.

A more effective technique for this nurse would have been formal intervention that the director could easily have initiated if she had known how to proceed. She would have had to: 1) list and document the professional practice problems, 2) document all behavioral observations related by the staff, and 3) document staff and patient complaints. Most of this information was already in hand. Significant colleagues could then have helped to present this information and their feelings about it to the nurse in a nonjudgmental, objective, caring way, expressing also their positive personal feelings for the nurse and their optimism about what treatment could offer. The director would then have encouraged the nurse to accept appropriate evaluation and whatever treatment would then be suggested.

In other words, in the scenario above, the data was there but the director wasn't sure how to use it. She had acted quite responsibly in spotting a problem, facing it, and insisting that steps be taken. There certainly was no absolute proof that the nurse was stealing Demerol, but there were ample clues that something was interfering with her ability to practice her profession. It's reasonable to expect responsible colleagues to **know** when there's a problem and to consider that alcohol/other drugs might well play a major part in it. But it's not necessary to know for a certainty **what** the problem is. That can be left to experts who when given full background information have both the ability to arrive at the correct diagnosis and the authority to report back on what the problem is and what should be done.

Where Do Colleagues Intervene?

Dealing with chemically dependent professionals demands flexibility and creativity in intervention planning, since their behavior is often unpredictable. No two situations are exactly alike, and personalities differ. Intervention specialists tell of interventions in parking lots, outside courthouses, in doctors' private offices (with patients sitting outside in the waiting room), in private homes, even in restaurants. (One of us has a fondness for the International House of Pancakes and Burger King and has successfully completed interventions in both!) Certainly the ideal situation is to hold the intervention in a quiet environment with full privacy while also not alerting the subject as to what will be taking place. Parish houses, law firms, university buildings, and hospitals have lots of meeting or conference rooms. The element of surprise is crucial so the person won't decide not to show up at all or won't have time to plan a defense strategy that may lead to turned tables and entrapment of the family or friends bent on successfully going through with an intervention. One pharmacist actually turned up at his own intervention with attorney in tow. Another brought along his psychologist, a kind, well-meaning but naive man convinced that continued analysis even in the face of active and worsening chemical dependence was the proper course of action.

Around the country some treatment programs are staffed with skilled intervenors. These specialists may be requested to travel to outlying areas to perform interventions. The actual **where** may not be determined until the intervenor arrives and attempts to catch up with the situation and then with the chemical dependent. A subject may sometimes be called to come to the intervenor's office under the guise of concerns expressed to the treatment program coordinator from anonymous persons regarding the subject's professional practice. He or she is invited to come and "straighten things out." Usually this is done in a very nonthreatening way so as not to alert the person to any threat or to hint that the visit is other than voluntary. A word of warning: If the intervenor is employed by a particular treatment center, he or she may have a vested interest in placing the patient at that facility, even if it's not in the best interest of the patient to go there.

Professional Intervention Programs

In recent years, the professions of law, pharmacy, medicine, dentistry, and nursing have acknowledged that some of their members are chemically dependent and have developed programs designed to help them. They fall into three types: 1) regulatory agency programs, 2) peer assistance programs, and 3) informal ("collegial") networks.

Regulatory Agency Programs

These programs (often called advocacy programs or rehabilitation programs) are moderated by state-level licensing boards and operate under state statutory guidelines. They may have a staff consultant with expertise in chemical dependence. The clear advantage of such programs is that impaired professionals who see their license endangered have a powerful incentive to cooperate with intervenors and accept treatment. However, **requiring** professions to report impaired or possibly impaired members (a procedure used in some states but not in others) calls forth strong arguments pro and con.

Those who favor obligatory reporting point out the obvious benefit mentioned above: that a threat to one's license motivates the professional to cooperate with intervenors and get treatment if necessary. Such a procedure, they say, saves not only the professional but the people he or she serves— people who might otherwise suffer serious harm. And they hold that in the absence of obligatory reporting, professional groups tend to be lax about reporting members who certainly need help.

Opponents object to the bureaucratic methods and set procedures of disciplinary committees of licensing boards. Moreover, they refer to obligatory reporting regulations as "snitch laws" and think of reporting their colleagues as an act of betrayal.

Some professional organizations advocate a two-tiered approach in which a nondisciplinary regulatory program first attempts early intervention and referral to treatment and turns the impaired professional over to a disciplinary board only if such attempts fail. They point out that the typical disciplinary board must follow rigid legal procedures that require a slow, thorough investigation and then a formal disciplinary hearing, so that the process may take well over a year. Meanwhile, they note, a professional who has been fired by an employer who has not notified the regulatory board of that action may continue active practice and retain full professional privileges, even though the alcohol/other drug use goes on, to the detriment of both the professional and the people he or she serves. Instead, these professional organizations say, they may well be able to conduct a swifter moving, less threatening early intervention that makes it unnecessary to take legal action or even to report the impaired professional for disciplinary action.

Peer Assistance Programs

The second type of program currently available for certain professions is a peer assistance program. Nursing, law, medicine, pharmacy, and dentistry have established many such programs through state professional associations and specialty groups. The most common type maintains a central office at a state association and has a cadre of trained intervenors in each of the state's regions. When a call for assistance is received, a coordinator contacts the closest intevenor to assist the person's supervisor, concerned colleague, or institution. Clearly, the disadvantage of a voluntary program is that it's voluntary. Over time it's difficult to maintain adequate staffing for this approach without funding and supportive services. Often these programs are manned only by volunteers, fellow professionals who already have time-consuming jobs, receive no compensation for their work, and often are provided no secretarial or clerical help, much less reimbursement for their time, travel expenses, and telephone bills. They've done a remarkable job in spite of these limitations, but a handful of concerned people can't be expected to meet the needs of hundreds of people scattered throughout a large state. Inevitably, calls for help will go unanswered or cases won't be given the time needed to do a thoughtful, thorough job. Peer assistance programs have had conflicts with regulatory agencies whose actions are sometimes arbitrary and insensitive. Some peer programs maintain adversarial relationships with the state in attempting to protect their members. However, in states with a regulatory-level program or committee, the two programs may work together to afford maximum support to the impaired professional while ensuring good care to clients or patients.

Informal ("Collegial") Networks

The third type of program is the least defined and yet is well established throughout the country. Informal or collegial networks exist in most large communities and are most often composed of people who also belong to 12-Step programs such as A.A. (Alcoholics Anonymous), or N.A. (Narcotics Anonymous). These programs include I.D.A.A. (International Doctors in A.A.), I.L.A.A. (International Lawyers in A.A.), L.C.L. (Lawyers Concerned for Lawyers), International Pharmacists Anonymous, International Nurses Anonymous, I.C.A.P. (Intercongregational Alcoholism Programs, for Catholic nuns), P.H.P. (Psychologists Helping Psychologists), S.W.H.S.W. (Social Workers Helping Social Workers), and many others.

Members of these programs are usually in recovery themselves and may serve as intervenors, but it's important to know that A.A. and similar groups don't themselves undertake any of these activities even though their individual members may do so. Some of the groups listed above will do so, but they generally don't use A.A. as part of their names. In general, these groups can be relied on to respect a newcomer's need for and right to anonymity. As groups, they don't make reports of any kind, and they use lists only to notify members of upcoming meetings or to do networking. Members of these groups have demonstrated a high personal degree of commitment in assisting their colleagues and are usually very effective in intervention, but of course they have limited leverage in intervention since they can share information with others only as members of other organizations and even then may not use confidences obtained through a mutual-help group.

There's indeed a place for the group that limits itself to advocacy and persuasion but doesn't in any way coerce. If a professional early in the disease process couldn't safely seek out information and explore whether there's even a problem, few would walk into a situation where the first admission of trouble would lead to a report to a disciplinary body.

The debate about which approach to use with impaired professional colleagues is silly, since this isn't an either/or situation. Both groups are needed, and needed simultaneously: those that move swiftly and coercively when necessary, and those that can be approached voluntarily, with full confidence that they can be trusted not to tattle or betray. Of course this means that at times members of voluntary groups will be profoundly uneasy as to what may happen to a colleague who's having problems. But if news gets out that voluntary groups can't keep a confidence, the word spreads rapidly, and persons who might otherwise come forward long before formal interventions are needed will be lost or can be dealt with only much later.

Peer-Initiated Intervention

Since the programs just described are already helping impaired professionals, why should you as a professional learn to intervene? The answer is simple: **You're needed**. For one thing, not every profession has its own programs. And many existing programs don't have the resources to help all those who need help; even the best of them are understaffed and short of funds. Medicine, for example, claims it has so-called "impaired" committees in every state, but some of them exist primarily on paper. What it boils down to, then, is that many a chemically dependent professional who desperately needs a caring, compassionate colleague to reach out and take the initiative in intervention that will pull him or her back from the brink of disaster simply gets no help. Then when a serious illness, accident, or even death strikes our colleague or his or her clients or patients, we wonder how we could have stood idly by and let it happen.

We need peer-initiated intervention to make up for the obvious limitations of regulatory programs. The big problem of regulatory programs is that they move too slowly—which often means too late. Because they often lack funds and hence sufficient personnel, they frequently have long waiting lists of professionals who have been reported and who need intervention and evaluation **now,** before they do further harm to themselves, their families, their trusting clients, and their profession. Another reason why regulatory programs move so slowly is that they must follow rigid procedures and weigh every bit of evidence. They tend to act only after a professional's deterioration is so obvious that charges brought against him or her can be proven. Their focus, then, isn't on early intervention but on monitoring treatment and recovery. But what we need is **early intervention**.

That's why we professionals need to learn about intervention and initiate it without delay (of course observing due process and showing real concern and respect) when we learn about the problems of an impaired colleague.

Chapter Highlights

In Chapter 3 we presented the basics of intervention:

Who: Any colleague who has concern and is willing to learn how to do an intervention.

What: Present the professional with significant data about his or her unacceptable professional practice or behavior.

When: When there's enough objective data about the professional's inability to practice safely because of apparent alcohol/other drug use.

Where: Any place that provides access to the professional and is nonthreatening.

We then identified several types of professional programs and discussed not only their advantages but their limitations. Limitations are:

- Regulatory agency programs (sponsored by licensing or certification boards): focus on discipline, treatment, monitoring, compliance; often lack resources for initiating intervention.
- Peer assistance programs (sponsored by professional associations, committees, or institutions): are traditionally voluntary, must depend on a small group of intervenors with limited time and resources.
- Informal (collegial) networks (often within 12-Step programs): lack professional leverage to encourage resisting professionals to accept treatment.

Part II

The Four Phases
of Intervention

Introduction to Part II

The chapters of Part II, summed up in the following chart, are based on a four-phase model for intervention: preparations (both initial and final—Chapters 4 and 5); actual intervention (Chapter 6); closure or resolution required of the intervenors, colleagues, and families (Chapter 7); and finally treatment and recovery (Chapter 8). The detailed stages in each of these phases follow a natural progression of interdependent events and should be observed without major changes.

The Four Phases of Intervention

1. Preparations:	*A. Initial*	*B. Final*
	Data Collection	Definition of Roles
	Selection of Team	Writing of Script
	Preparation of Team	Ground Rules
	Action Plan	Rehearsal
	Handling	
	of Team's Anxieties	
2. Intervention:	Use of Leverage	
	Safety Precautions	
	Wrapping Up	
3. Closure:	Needs of Team	
	Dealing with Co-workers, Families	
	Taking Care of You	
4. Treatment and Recovery:	Evaluation	
	Treatment	
	Recovery Issues	
	Monitoring	

Chapter 4

Phase One:
Initial Preparations

Because intervention is a highly integrated team process, there must be a designated leader or coordinator. This may be a colleague, a friend, a supervisor, or an advocate representing a peer assistance program or regulatory board. If you want to become the leader, you should meet these criteria: 1) You're willing to accept the responsibility for doing it thoughtfully and well; 2) you have genuine concern for the chemically dependent professional; and 3) you'll follow the guidelines for intervention as presented in this book and/or will receive training in intervention techniques. We know that other resources for peer intervention within our professions, employment settings, and communities remain very limited. So the ultimate goal of this book is to prepare you to assume the role of the intervention coordinator yourself or at least to be an active and useful participant. **From this point on, we'll be speaking to you as the colleague who's also the coordinator.** If others are willing to read and learn along with you, all to the good.

The first task in preparing to intervene with a chemically dependent colleague is deciding who will do what when and how. You may be the one who first became aware of the problem, or the one who received reports from colleagues; but regardless of how you became involved, you've already made two crucial decisions: that action is needed, and that you're willing to become involved. The role of the coordinator resembles that of the conductor of a symphony who selects the score to be performed and trains a variety of instrumentalists to play together to achieve the sound of a full orchestra. Although each of these musicians may individually possess artistic excellence, no soloist can produce the rich sound of a Beethoven symphony. This is equally true of intervention. In a nutshell, the coordinator's role is to select and prepare people who care about a chemically dependent professional and who can work together to present, in an acceptable way, their concerns and feelings about that person's alcohol/other drug use.

In Phase One, the first of your specific functions as coordinator is to see to the collection of data.

Collecting the Data

Collecting data is the meat of the matter. While this procedure isn't as dramatic as the intervention itself, your effectiveness in the intervention will depend greatly on how thorough a job you do now. Unless you've gathered appropriate data, you may not have down-to-earth, hard facts that will be strong enough to counteract the chemical dependent's denial of even (to you) very visible and serious professional or personal problems.

Data collection actually begins on an almost subconscious level. Something or someone alerts us in some small way that a certain colleague might have a problem. We usually don't first think of alcohol/other drugs on a conscious level; we attribute the subtle changes to some other plausible cause: "He's going through that tough divorce and trying to prepare for boards," "She's working full-time and trying to handle those kids," "She's really been down since her mother died," and so on. Regardless of how successfully we rationalize these warning signs, little hints about the possibility of an alcohol/other drug problem remain in our memories. Meanwhile, others are reacting much as we do. They may even have mentioned their observations to us and to others, asking, "Have you noticed anything unusual about Ed?" or "Is something going on?"

Once our antennae are up, we begin not only to notice but to assess exactly what **is** going on. As in any professional situation where we need to collect information before taking action, we collect pieces of data that we feel will help us get a better picture. Data collection for intervention is exactly that: a methodical assessment of a chemical dependent's professional functioning. We're familiar with the art of assessment as practiced daily in our own field and are usually able to adapt our skills to a variety of persons and settings. Through practice we've gained the expertise that allows us to be flexible and creative in our assessments, to track down clues that lead us to a satisfactory result. It helps if we think of data collection as a process, sometimes rather a long one, rather than a single event. The actual steps follow logically.

Let's illustrate from the field of medicine. There's a natural flow in assessing possible illness: a chief complaint or symptom, medical/surgical history, psychiatric history, current medical conditions, family/social history, and occupational information. In certain medical specialties the emphasis is on tracking down causes. If we suspect infectious disease, for example, we want to know about any recent travel so we can learn of possible exposure to certain bacteria or parasites, or about sexual practices and experiences when we're considering the possibility of sexually transmitted diseases.

So data collection is already common and familiar. We all do it. In preparing to do an intervention, we just have to change the focus from medical illness, pastoral counseling, or preparing a court case—or whatever our field is—to a problem that has its roots in dependence on alcohol/other drugs. To illustrate the parallels, we'll compare the data collection phase of intervention to medical assessment, pointing out six analogous features.

Medical Assessment/Collecting Intervention Data

Medical Model	*Intervention Model*
1. Chief complaint	1. Precipitating event
2. Medical/surgical history	2. Professional performance
3. Psychiatric history	3. Interpersonal relations
4. Current medical conditions	4. Medical/physical complications
5. Family/social history	5. Family/social changes
6. Occupational information	6. Legal data

Here, one by one, are the six parallels:

1. (Medical Field:) Chief Complaint
(Intervention:) Precipitating Event

In every case of intervention, a crisis or incident triggered something that started the process. Something occurred for the first time or happened once too often, and someone decided it was time to do something. The person reporting the information may be a client, a policeman, a patient, a student, or a colleague such as a law partner, a staff nurse or physician or pharmacist; or it may be a friend or family member or even a casual observer. But someone gave information to someone who should be told. This precipitating event is the equivalent of the medical "chief complaint." Something is wrong with someone for some reason. The information tentatively offered or indignantly dumped on that someone else with the expectation that something will be done varies with the situation. It may be "He came in drunk again," "She went to sleep at lunchtime in the lounge, and we couldn't wake her up," "Another failure to file," "He forgot which patients were his and wrote the wrong orders," "The Demerol count is off again, and she signed out three doses on the same patient." Regardless of the complaint, there's always some final precipitating event—something that gets the ball rolling.

While serving as consultant to the Board of Nursing in Florida, one of us got a call from a staff nurse in a northern Florida hospital who stated there was an impaired nurse on the night shift whose supervisor refused to do anything about her condition. The nurse allegedly came to work smelling of alcohol and often interrupted the oral report being given by the off-going shift with demands that things be repeated. Several times other staff had observed her sleeping at the nurses' station, but their reports brought no action. The Director of Nursing was told of the complaint. She seemed very concerned and agreed to investigate. Soon she called back, stating she had found the nurse asleep on duty and smelling of alcohol. The immediate supervisor had been protecting this nurse, who had young children and financially couldn't afford to lose her job. The supervisor's enabling had of course only delayed discovery. The staff nurse who called to report the situation provided the precipitating event.

2. (Medical Field:)   Medical/Surgical History
(Intervention:)   Professional Performance

As we collect data in order to assess changes in a professional's behavior, we must have a baseline, a standard against which we can measure those changes. That is, we need to know the history of that person's **usual** performance before these recent changes and how that performance was regarded by colleagues, supervisors, clients, patients. An important source of a person's professional performance is written records. Such records are immensely important because they're objective. There are the facts, in black and white, with no tint or taint of personal opinion or prejudice, pro or con. Written records can answer such crucial questions as these: Have there ever been disciplinary warnings or conferences about poor performance? Any unusual occurrences, errors, or accidents? A pattern of absenteeism or frequent illness? Or the reverse, a refusal to take vacations or time off? Recent errors of judgment?

The following chart focuses on six kinds of records available for collecting data about the performance of healthcare professionals. Inspecting records might reveal, for example, suspicious discrepancies between the amount of drugs supposedly on hand and the amount administered to patients, or between what a patient actually received and what the nurse supposedly administered. **But this healthcare chart can be adapted to many other professions,** since all professions have written records of some kind. A close look at almost any kind of written records—a lawyer's legal briefs or a client's records, notes taken down by a counselor at a counseling session, notes of a clergyperson's planned sermon or a teacher's lecture—might reveal uncharacteristic illogical, incoherent thinking that signals serious problems.

Collecting Data from Records of Healthcare Professionals

1. Narcotics
   A. Discrepancies in sign-out sheets
   B. Wastages (following procedures for proper discarding of unused drugs, and documentation of witnessed discarding)
   C. Supply records (stock)—amounts, frequency of order
2. Medication records
   A. Doses recorded accurately
   B. Correspond with notes and narcotic records as to the amount or drug given
3. Progress notes/nurses' notes/records
   A. Appropriate
   B. Complete
   C. Legible

4. Doctor's orders
   A. Appropriate
   B. Written for correct patient
   C. Complete
5. Anesthesia records/surgical records
   A. Medication orders—recorded and appropriate
   B. Documentation—recorded and appropriate
   C. Post-op orders
6. Legal/professional records
   A. Work history in prior positions
   B. Disciplinary actions by employer or licensing board
   C. Incident reports (errors or accidents involving the subject)
   D. Attendance records
   E. DUI/DWI charges

The following incident illustrates how helpful it can be to review records.

To help a community hospital director review records in collecting data for possible intervention on a 30-year-old male nurse, we requested all the narcotic records from that unit for the current month and the two previous months. The current month sign-out sheet for Demerol was what precipitated the intervention process. It contained several occurrences of "wastages" of large amounts of Demerol by this nurse, with no cosignatures. Also, a staff member had reported that the nurse was spending a great deal of time in the bathroom and acting "spaced out" at times. The record of Demerol sign-outs was a red light! Not only had he "wasted" whole tubexes of Demerol, but his name appeared more often than any other. Records of the two preceding months showed similar wastages and missing cosignatures. Over the three-month period, this nurse "wasted" approximately 1600 mg of Demerol. Obviously no one had reviewed the completed narcotic records before they were sent to the pharmacy.

In this case the records alone provided the bulk of the data needed for intervention. Also, when several cosignatures that did exist on some of his "wastes" were checked, they had ostensibly been written by nurses who weren't on duty that day. Several patient records were pulled to cross-check the doses signed out. These charts indicated no administration of Demerol. Several of the patients who had Demerol signed out in their names were never ordered Demerol by the physician.

When a physician is suspected of diversion, reviewing hospital pharmacy records can be very enlightening. Does he or she get office narcotics from the pharmacy? How frequently? Has the ordering increased recently? How about "personal prescriptions"? Also, many of the large drugstore chains now have computer access to prescriptions in all other branches of their stores and can pull up those lists according to the physician's name. In private practice, whether with people or animals, if controlled drugs are used, they may be ordered by office staff. If the drugs are being diverted, there will be more frequent and/or larger orders of stock. Such discrepancies are excellent data for the intervention and will help us document our impressions.

A staff physician in a community hospital reported to the physician peer assistance coordinator that a good friend of his, also a staff physician, had asked him to sign a prescription for Demerol tablets, allegedly for a girlfriend with long-standing medical problems requiring pain medication. The doctor asking for the signature explained that he had been writing too many prescriptions and that the pharmacy was getting suspicious. The doctor did sign the prescription and entered his DEA (Drug Enforcement Agency) number but never actually saw the patient. In the medical staff lounge he casually mentioned this episode to another physician, also a good friend, who said, "You too!" Apparently three other staff physicians had been asked for prescriptions for Demerol, and, surprisingly, all had signed them. The pharmacy had significant documentation of very frequent ordering of stock narcotics for this doctor's office, and other local pharmacies were refusing to fill any more prescriptions over his signature.

In our review of records we also might examine the work history if employment applications and resumés are available. Persons who have been in a certain geographic location only a short time often leave a problem behind. Many professionals are still in great demand and can easily run from a difficult situation to a new location. Many report that they never were fired or even reprimanded but that when their work deteriorated and they sensed that the axe was about to fall, they resigned. In most cases the employers seemed pleased not to have to deal with the situation and often went on to write flattering letters of recommendation. Some employers say they're afraid not to write such letters because they're afraid of litigation if they report something that might be seen as damaging. However, it would be naive to focus on only relatively new employees. For example, the majority of nurse referrals for chemical dependence problems over a two-year period in the Tampa Program were hospital employees of two years or more.

The recently mentioned nurse who was discovered through review of narcotic records had been employed at the hospital for approximately a year. He had moved to Florida from another Southern state, where he had actually once admitted to diverting Demerol and had been terminated for that reason. Unfortunately that hospital never filed a complaint with the Board of Nursing, preferring to act as if it hadn't known the facts. The nurse was quite properly granted a license to practice in Florida, since there was no mention of disciplinary action on his record. He came to Florida intending to start over (an attempt at the proverbial "geographic cure" so often mentioned by chemical dependents in recovery) but didn't realize his problem would inevitably follow him. By the time of his intervention in Florida he had been diverting Demerol regularly for over three years.

Legal/disciplinary records (see # 6 in the preceding chart) are most helpful in revealing a person's current professional status—and knowing that status is important in helping you determine your options and your leverage. It's important to know whether a person has already had a license suspended, been warned, or been placed on probation, because such disciplinary action may drastically affect your ability to offer reprieve from further punishment. Many states define in their professional practice act the conditions under which a professional may receive discipline, what type of discipline it must be, and how many times a board's disciplinary action may occur before a license is permanently revoked. Some states also control criteria for admission to a state-level peer assistance program; those criteria include never having been subjected to disciplinary action for chemical abuse. If the professional you're dealing with has had such prior disciplinary action, has had a license reinstated, and is now again in violation of the state's professional practice act, you may not be able to offer enrollment in a regulatory program in lieu of board action. This determination is central to evaluating what leverage you have and what the focus of the leverage will be. If you can't offer disciplinary immunity, perhaps the enticement to enter treatment and receive aftercare must be limited to the hope of reducing the time of suspension imposed by the board.

Sometimes the professional is currently under investigation from a previous complaint, but this information is considered privileged until a hearing is held and board action taken. The disciplinary process in most states takes well over a year from first report to final fruition: the full investigation and completed board hearing. When the initial report is filed with the licensing board, the professional is frequently terminated from the place of employment but usually secures immediate employment elsewhere. The new employer will be unaware of the investigation, and the professional may even omit a mention of the last employer from the resumé, giving an excuse to explain why there's a time gap in the employment history. Such excuses are particularly easy for women, whose responsibilities for children or household often make a short hiatus from work desirable. Serious illness or death in the family are also popular explanations, as is the need for a few weeks or months in which to write a book. Since many books are never completed or never accepted, there's no need to produce an actual book to make this excuse plausible.

Each state department of professional regulation has as its primary goal to protect the public from inadequately trained, unsafe, and unethical professionals. These departments employ investigators to follow up on complaints about licensed professionals from employers, colleagues, and the public. If the professional is already under investigation, that investigation may be used to advantage. It's sometimes possible to involve the investigator assigned to the case. Many such investigators have extensive background not only in regulatory monitoring but also in statutory procedure and can help you prepare leverage. In some communities where there are clearly identified advocacy groups for professionals, the investigators may call the peer assistance coordinators and request help in intervention. Many of the investigators we have dealt with have a commitment not only to collecting evidence to make a case against someone but also to really helping those who need help.

Too often we see the regulatory board and its extensions only as the enemy, but this can work to our disadvantage. These groups vary a great deal from state to state and system to system; some are excellent. The persons who work in investigative divisions are often very competent and eager to assess accurately the alleged situation and to present it objectively to the regulatory agency. Although they're not obligated to help, many have attempted to identify community treatment resources for the chemically dependent professional and sometimes even initiate the contact. This doesn't mean that the investigative process won't continue, but it does mean that there's an opportunity to receive treatment. This, after all, meets the primary goal of all concerned: promoting safety for the public and recovery for the professional. Their offer of help isn't entirely altruistic, since disciplinary bodies are often overburdened and backlogged. If they can find ways to help people move out of practice and into treatment rapidly, the more enlightened ones can see this as much more desirable than going through the long, tedious, painful, expensive disciplinary process.

Unfortunately, some measure success only by the total number of scalps collected and convictions secured. But we repeat: Not all states and all professions are alike. What's available and useful in one location may be just the opposite in another. Some regulatory agency staffs are eager to help rather than punish. Others seem bent on demolishing any professional who they can prove has broken a law, and they'll wreak vengeance on people even years after a successful recovery has taken place.

Please take time to learn in advance what the situation really is in your own bar association, dental society, or other professional organization, as well as the operating procedures of your own governmental disciplinary agencies before deciding how and when to involve them. Know what the law requires you to do, and be aware of your options before you take action.

3. (Medical Field:)   Psychiatric History
(Intervention:)   Interpersonal Relations

This third area of data collection focuses on changes in behavior and interactions with others that can be noted in the professional environment. A relatively rare, isolated instance of any of these behaviors may not be significant, but when they accumulate so much that they become a **pattern** of behavior, they mustn't be ignored as indicators of chemical dependence, even though they involve personal judgment more than perusing written records does. **(Please note that these indicators apply to professionals in any field.)**

Collecting Behavioral Data on Impaired Professionals

1. Unusual behavior while at work
2. Inappropriate behavior toward
   A. Staff
   B. Clients or patients
   C. Colleagues
3. Mood swings
4. Poor judgment
5. Declining quality of performance
6. Decline in physical appearance and personal grooming
7. Increase in physical complaints
8. Frequent physical or emotional illness

9. Withdrawal from friends, colleagues
10. Change in usual work schedule
    A. Frequently late
    B. Always at work
    C. "Visits" on days off
    D. Schedule erratic/unpredictable
    E. Blackouts
11. Physical symptoms caused by alcohol/other drug use
    A. Tremors/twitching
    B. Profuse perspiration
    C. Pupils dilated/constricted

The impaired person will go through subtle personality changes as the disease progresses and may one day seem to have become someone totally different from the person you once knew. Often there are mood swings, perhaps seen in irritability, outbursts of anger, sudden euphoria, hyperactivity, or paranoia. Other staff may have noticed these behavioral changes and often will discuss with each other that someone is "awfully touchy lately," "is getting cranky a lot," or seems "pretty down." If possible, several of these observers should record the events exactly as they occurred, noting the nature of the interaction, who was involved, who witnessed the situation, and the date and time of each occurrence. Staff members usually have more than enough information for any one intervention, but comments in isolation are often disregarded. In collecting your data, learn which staff have the most interaction with the person being investigated; often they will already have complained or voiced their concern to someone.

If the person is under the influence while on duty, other observations might be documented. Of course major outbursts or gruffness with clients or patients are easily recognized as inappropriate, but here we're referring to actions clearly out of step with the context in which they are performed. Some impaired physicians make rounds at 2 a.m., waking up patients and disrupting staff routine. One California surgeon had a T-shirt saying "Midnight

Marauder" that he said was given to him because of when he made rounds. One wonders! Other physicians may not respond while "on call" for emergencies, so others must be called in.

Disorientation does occur because of certain drugs. As a result, the person may reach for things that aren't there, have significant memory lapses, report for duty on the wrong day, forget to come to work at all when scheduled, have inappropriate conversations with clients, patients, or visitors, or "nod off" while talking to a client or writing charts. All of this behavior should be documented by those who observe it. The impaired person may have no memory of much of it, so presenting it during an intervention can have a profound effect.

A 27-year-old nurse working in a small community hospital was reported to peer assistance as "acting strangely." The staff stated that she appeared "sort of out of it" and on several occasions rambled on and on in ways that made no sense. After consultation with the director, the night supervisor was asked to monitor the situation for several weeks. During this time, the nurse told the supervisor that everyone was out to get her. The staff noticed that when her patients required injections for pain, she administered the medications but saved all the dirty syringes in her pocket. When she was questioned about this, she became extremely hostile and defensive. During this several weeks, she had made several significant errors in transcribing doctors' orders, and these errors were documented in incident reports. Because of these documented events and a sudden unprovoked temper tantrum, it was recommended that the director and supervisor prepare for intervention immediately. During the intervention a urine sample was requested from the nurse, which she gave willingly. Her drug screen showed positive for three major classifications of drugs.

This nurse had been employed at another community hospital, where she had diverted numerous patient medications and had been referred to a psychiatrist as a possible suicide risk. Fearing rejection, she hadn't told her employer all the places where she had worked.

The marked changes in her behavior served as excellent data for detecting professional performance problems. When she was questioned after the intervention about keeping the old syringes in her pocket, she said she was so paranoid about diverting drugs that she lived in constant fear that someone would ask her if she had really given her patients their medication. She thought that if she could produce some physical evidence such as the syringes, it would prove she had.

4. (Medical Field:)   Current Medical Conditions
(Intervention:)   Medical/Physical Complications

Many people suffer medical consequences from their alcohol/other drug use. Knowing their health status is an excellent adjunct to the other data we're collecting. In institutional settings there are three valuable sources of such information: 1) Employee Health Services, 2) emergency-room staff and records in hospitals, and 3) personnel records that note absenteeism, allegedly for illness, or that have doctors' notes attesting to these illnesses.

The emergency room in any hospital frequently is used almost as a family doctor's office; staff are treated there for a variety of minor complaints as well as in true emergency situations. The person dependent primarily on alcohol may suffer blackouts and repeated minor accidents. More serious accidents may involve other persons who have been injured as well, and all the victims may be treated in the emergency room. Even when injuries don't require hospitalization, the word goes out on the hospital grapevine, and there's little secret about who was there and why. Additionally, there may be other accidents at home leading to the emergency room for a range of problems, from falls to other variously explained cuts, burns, sprains, or fractures.

Black eyes, almost always attributed to having been mugged or to a collision with a door or cabinet, aren't uncommon in professional women who are chemically dependent and are abused by husbands or boyfriends— men who may themselves be heavy drinkers or users. People dependent on injectable narcotics have seizures due to drug toxicity, particularly if they're taking large amounts of Demerol. Cocaine users do so as well, just as alcoholics and other sedative addicts may have seizures when they're not using and are, in fact, having seizures that aren't from the toxicity caused by excessive use but that are a sign of withdrawal.

If these people work in hospitals and are on duty at the time, they're usually brought at once to the emergency room. They probably won't volunteer their history of alcohol/other drug use, and unless it's already suspected, medical professionals treating them will ultimately explain most of these episodes as seizures of unknown origin or as idiopathic epilepsy. As a result, many alcoholics are taking unneeded Dilantin (a drug used to control seizures).

Opiate drug users and others who inject their drugs may develop abscesses at injection sites but may not seek attention until the abscesses are quite advanced and painful. They may seek treatment far from the work site, but even if they do, two problems remain: 1) identifying the source of the abscess as drug-related, and 2) recognizing the drug-seeking behavior of the chemical dependent who's asking for pain medicine. When questioned about the abscesses, chemical dependents usually have an elaborate explanation to explain the infection. Healthcare workers may limit their self-injection to muscles and to lower extremities, so there are often no visible "tracks" over arm veins.

A young intern working on a pediatric surgical unit was using I.V. Demerol. She had poor veins and had used her arm veins so frequently for injections of narcotics and cocaine that they were scarred, occluded, and could no longer be used. She began injecting drugs into her feet and developed a significant abscess and cellulitis (an infection) of the right foot. The foot became so swollen that she was limping and couldn't tie her shoe. One evening at work an attending physician insisted she go with him to the emergency room to be examined. There her greatest fear was that someone would know how she had developed the cellulitis. To her mind one would have to be blind to miss the injection sites. When the physician there, a surgeon, asked how she had developed this condition, she said, "A chair dropped on my foot." He asked no further questions but treated and discharged her after writing a prescription for antibiotics and pain medications. The incident was never mentioned again.

Whether the physician did recognize the signs of her drug use, the point is that we tend to accept or pretend to accept the explanation that creates the least conflict for us. No one wants to think of a colleague as a chemical dependent or even to suspect it. Even if we do suspect it, we tend to shrug it off by asking ourselves what we can do without creating a big hassle for all concerned.

Although most healthcare professionals have some opportunity to divert drugs from the office or hospital, some continue their pattern of drug seeking wherever there's a possibility of obtaining a more legitimate supply. Those in other professions must turn to the street or to someone else to prescribe. Such people are often seen in emergency rooms with vague or even specific subjective complaints requiring pain prescriptions. Some of them frequent doctors' offices and employee health services requesting prescriptions; or what's even easier, hospital staff obtain prescriptions from other doctors or other staff in hallways, in the cafeteria, or while they're making rounds. If prescriptions are filled in the hospital pharmacy, though, records may easily be obtained. If a number of different pharmacies are used and particularly if the drug of choice doesn't require a triplicate prescription (a special form required in some states for obtaining certain mind-altering drugs), this becomes more difficult. If the addiction is to a benzodiazapine, such as Valium, which is prescribed very casually, the task is even harder.

Another possible source is the dentist's office, where it's standard protocol to offer patients pain medication after certain dental procedures—not an unusual way for people to be introduced to the effects of narcotics.

In short, drug-seeking behavior, when suspected, asked about, and documented, provides extremely valuable data, particularly if it can be described in writing.

Employee Health Services are an additional source of medical data, but information kept there is normally confidential. There have nonetheless been situations where suspected chemical dependents were reported to administrative staff by the employee health nurse, whose records provided excellent documentation for intervention. In some situations, interventions have been performed in the employee health department itself.

A 30-year-old nurse employed in a large teaching hospital was referred to the Employee Health Services after coming to work nauseated, pale, and tremulous. This nurse had recently been sent for counseling because of increasing absenteeism, and the head nurse felt that because of her still-frequent call-ins and current condition, she should be evaluated. Also, a staff member on the off-going shift reported to the head nurse that she had smelled alcohol on this nurse's breath that same morning—not the first such episode. The nurse went to the Employee Health Services (EHS) that morning and saw the nurse practitioner, who after her initial assessment called the local peer assistance program stating she felt the nurse was intoxicated and that she wasn't sure how to proceed. It was recommended that she draw a blood alcohol and obtain a urine screen with the nurse's permission. The nurse agreed to both tests and to resting in EHS while waiting for the doctor. In the meantime the peer assistance committee mobilized rapidly, collected the background data from the head nurse's well-documented material on the recent absenteeism and performance issues, and met with the nurse practitioner, Director of Nursing, and a personnel staff member in the conference room at the EHS. With adequate data collected to demonstrate the nurse's decline in performance, increasing absenteeism, and the present odor of alcohol on her breath, intervention was initiated within one hour of the phone call. During the intervention the nurse admitted, "I've been drinking a little too much" and agreed to an evaluation in order to protect her job.

When her parents arrived to drive her home they expressed heartfelt gratitude to the members of the intervention team because they saw the hospital as rescuing their child. They had thought that if the hospital found out, she would simply be fired. It evidently had never occurred to them that any other approach would be used.

Another source of medical information is the primary physician, who may often identify a problem with a healthcare professional but not really be sure what to do about it. You may be the confidant the physician chooses to help determine what course to follow. Of course, the primary physician has records of medical findings and other indications of alcohol/other drug use but may lack a clear perspective on other possibly dysfunctional areas of a patient's professional practice and family life. Without these other pieces of information to confirm suspicions, a physician may believe the usual excuses, rationalizations, and denial that obscure the necessity for intervention. However, the ideal situation for intervention using medical data includes the primary-care physician, who participates as an active team member and presents concerns in the context of the person's physical health. In cases of advanced alcoholism, for example, there may be significant demonstrable liver involvement. Other common findings are those of essential hypertension and glucose intolerance. These objective signs are excellent tools for a practitioner to use in intervention. Of course, these approaches will always be complicated by considerations of confidentiality, but when confidentiality conflicts with the person's need for treatment, ways can often be devised to honor both. (One possibility is to have the primary physician present at the onset of the intervention and to ask the patient for permission to mention medical findings, a request that's usually granted.)

5. (Medical Field:)   Family/Social History
(Intervention:)   Family/Social Changes

An important part of any thorough assessment is the family/social history. We evaluate the individual in relation both to the larger social environment and to the risk factors for illness within the family system. In medicine there are certain classifications of disease in which genetic risk-factor assessment is routine, as in heart disease, high blood pressure, and diabetes. Chemical dependence should be another. In collecting the data for intervention, family/social changes as a result of the alcohol/other drug use are important, although the family history of chemical dependence is often not obtained until treatment is under way. However, it helps to be aware of the person's significant family and other relationships and any personal conflicts that may have occurred recently. There are predictable disruptions, since chemical dependence usually begins to affect home and personal relationships first (the area of professional practice is most often the last to be affected). Important data is bound to be there and sometimes will be readily available.

In some cases, trying to get information about a person's personal relationships is counterproductive. Many impaired people will long since have lost roommates or family and now live alone. If the work site provides adequate material, and particularly if one has the real clout of being able to threaten a person's license to practice, family data may not be as important in this type of intervention. If on the other hand the colleague is retired, works alone, or is in a profession where little if anything is done to regulate professional behavior, threats to interfere with the practice are really little more than hot air. The family's involvement is then essential.

Obviously one wants to avoid stirring up rumors and destructive gossip about a colleague, but a little reflection may suggest reasonable places to look further. Were you formerly a good friend of both members of a couple now divorced? Did you ever hear from the former spouse what really happened? Did you even want to know at the time? This may be the time to get in touch with that person and find out.

By the time we begin collecting work-related data, many of our sick colleagues will have suffered severe personal losses, and many of these losses are common knowledge among their colleagues. Frequently a recent separation or a child in trouble with drugs is presented by other professionals as the reason for rather than the result of the heavy drinking or using, particularly if the drugs are tranquilizers or other sedatives. As we discussed earlier, professionals who are members of law firms, social-work agencies, or hospital staffs often function like extended families, particularly when the same people work together a long time. So we know more about each other than we think. When you look for it, you'll find that much family and personal information is common knowledge.

Also, there will be information to gather regarding changes in the person's significant relationships with others on the job. The chemically dependent person usually gets busy with other things and slowly withdraws as the disease progresses. Those who have been close friends feel their colleague pulling away, and their old shared activities often stop altogether. Many times colleagues when asked whether they still see the person socially will say, "We used to see each other often, but lately she always has something else to do or doesn't feel like going out." Or you might hear, "Our work group always goes out Fridays after work, but he hasn't been coming lately."

Professionals who are part of small or individual practices may have a group of colleagues with whom they socialize. They might have breakfast meetings with other clergy, faculty-club functions, a card game at someone's home. Even long-standing office relationships have many of the same qualities as family relationships, and changes in these are important to understand. Office staff often have lots of valuable intervention documentation, though getting them to share it is sometimes difficult. A loyal secretary can be a fiercer defender than many a wife.

In assessing significant personal and professional relationships we're really looking for two things: 1) How much personal loss, if any, has the person already suffered from the chemical dependence? and 2) is he or she on the verge of losing something or someone else very important? First, then, knowing about recent changes in family status gives perspective on the progression of the disease and any losses already undergone. This is critical not only when trying to decide the most effective leverage for intervention but also in assessing the risk of suicide after intervention. We'll discuss this later in more detail. It's important to be aware of particularly destructive living arrangements, such as a woman living with a wife beater or an alcoholic girlfriend. Secondly, if spouse, children, and home aren't yet lost, there may be some further leverage for the intervention. (In some instances, family members who have left specifically because they can no longer tolerate the alcohol/other drug-related behavior may still want to help. An alienated spouse may even reconsider a reconciliation if the intervention succeeds and is followed by stable recovery.) Spouses may have to be included in a professional intervention if they're an essential part of the leverage to be used. Often, spouses and significant others are the ones who initiate the request for help; they can provide invaluable data to the intervention team even if it's decided it's best for them not to participate in the intervention itself. In spite of our earlier warnings about including them, at times no other way is likely to work, and the risk must be taken. The key is to assess thoroughly their ability to participate.

The wife of a pharmacist working at a large teaching hospital in Texas asked him to call a peer assistance program to get help with his drinking problem. When he did call, he minimized his drinking, stating that it hadn't interfered with his work but that his wife was concerned, quite unnecessarily. Later, his wife told of numerous episodes of his uncontrolled drinking, threatening behavior, and even some actual violence. He was unpredictable, and when he was drinking his rage frightened her and their two-year-old. He was unreasonably possessive of her, accused her of infidelity, and tracked her every move. His days off were spent at home drinking. When hangovers were bad or he was too drunk to go to work, she called in for him and made excuses. She was expecting a second child and had threatened to leave him unless things changed. She meant it.

After this conversation the pharmacist's peer assistance coordinator met with the wife, and together they planned a formal intervention. The pharmacist hadn't understood how serious his wife's threats to leave him were. During the intervention, his colleagues clearly explained that they expected him to admit himself to a chemical dependence treatment center. He agreed, and his wife agreed to stay and see what would happen. While in treatment he realized that he was indeed alcoholic, and he told his employer that he was in treatment and why. His position was held for him, and he was placed on sick leave until his discharge from treatment.

Clearly, his wife's ultimatum was the only thing that had moved him to get help. Interestingly, after the employer was notified and the pharmacist had signed release forms that the peer assistance program could work with his employer to plan for his return to work, the employer and the peer assistance program identified several other problem areas in his job performance other than the absenteeism. After the pharmacist had told other staff what had happened to him, one staff member admitted that she had smelled alcohol on his breath several times when he reported on duty but had never mentioned it to anyone. The clues were there, but no one had put the picture together and acted on it. Had his wife not been firm in her demands, he might have continued working and drinking until some serious, perhaps fatal, accident had happened. (He often drank before driving a fifty-mile round trip to and from work.)

Although our experience has been that friends and family report relatively few professionals to peer assistance programs, those who recognize the problem and are committed to helping the person get treatment can be powerful allies in the intervention process.

6. (Medical Field:)   Occupational Information
(Intervention:)   Legal Data

Sometimes legal entanglements indicate chemical dependence. For instance, Driving Under the Influence (DUI) episodes, often reduced to reckless driving, are important documentation for intervention. It's important to realize that only a tiny percentage of those who drive after heavy drinking are ever arrested. The odds against this happening are so great (in some areas less than one in every 500) that if a person is arrested more than once, many experts feel that this reflects perhaps more than 1000 actual trips made while under the influence. If two arrests can be documented for someone who is already suspected of being alcoholic, there's little chance that the concern of colleagues is exaggerated.

Many states now have formal programs for DUI/DWI offenses that require the offender to attend state-sponsored educational counseling sessions. Some professionals do go through these programs, but their affluence, sophistication, and ability to hire attorneys make this much less likely than for many others. Women are even less likely to be booked, much less convicted, for DUI than men. One social worker said she had actually been stopped several times, but "I'd just cry a little for the officer and talk about my babies and their sitter waiting at home." Another, a nun, said she had been pulled over repeatedly but that as soon as the arresting officer saw her habit, that ended any question of arrest. Twice she was driven home by one officer while his partner followed in the patrol car.

These programs are no substitute for treatment if the people arrested are alcoholics rather than merely irresponsible drinkers. The counseling these programs offer is very limited. Although professionals can often buy their way out of a DUI charge, those who find themselves in mandatory DUI education sessions are often surrounded by young laypeople from whom it's all too easy to disassociate themselves ("I'm not like those people"). The DUI arrests and sessions do provide a form of early intervention that's sometimes effective, but only rarely. However, one young woman medical student was sent by the court for private counseling to an excellent alcoholism counselor who referred her to an A.A. group with which she was entirely comfortable. Some communities have excellent links between the court system and peer assistance programs and may notify peer assistance coordinators of healthcare professionals who are convicted of DUI offenses. These convictions are a matter of public record, so no confidentiality is violated. Also, some newspapers routinely report police actions within the community, and the professional may be publicly exposed, although in urban areas colleagues are usually unaware of such arrests and learn of them only after deliberately pursuing information.

The chemically dependent professional may be named in litigation for malpractice or in other lawsuits related to alcohol/other drug use. Determining whether the legal problem is related to such use may be difficult, but if it is and if you have documentation to support your position, it's advisable to contact the professional's attorney. Try to enlist the attorney's support for the planned intervention and for the evaluation/treatment that is the goal of the intervention team. Realize, though, that because some attorneys, like other professionals, know little about chemical dependence, you may encounter resistance. Some attorneys will see their client's acceptance of evaluation/ treatment as tantamount to admitting chemical dependence; they fear that any such supposed admission will bolster the accusations of those who initiated the litigation. On the other hand, some attorneys will see that voluntarily seeking evaluation/treatment may give substance to their client's statements of good intentions and assertions that he or she is working on the problem. Realize, too, that attorneys will look carefully at how accepting evaluation/ treatment will probably affect the outcome of each kind of trial. For instance, accepting it may be a real asset for the client in a child-custody case but may be a liability in a malpractice suit, where it may be pounced on as a confession of guilt.

The preceding walk-through of the data-collection process shows that it really isn't so difficult. Notice, we don't focus on alcohol/other drug use itself but on behavioral manifestations of it, particularly in professional practice. The exact number of drinks taken, capsules swallowed, or lines snorted is no more important than knowing how many bacteria are involved in a case of pneumonia. What's important is what alcohol/other drugs or those bacteria are doing. If we focus on proving "inappropriate" use of alcohol/other drugs we may be endangering the whole intervention. How many drinks are too many, and how do we prove it? It takes a long time to collect this sort of proof. We don't need it, and we may lose the battle during intervention if the subject insists he or she didn't take a particular drug on that particular occasion.

When we focus on collecting accurate and complete data related to matters of professional practice, however, we're on more solid ground and can ignore some of the necessary ego defenses ("I'm not an addict" or "I'm not an alcoholic"). We don't need to know exactly what or how many drinks or other drugs were used, and we leave the gradual dismantling of denial to the treatment team after we've done our part and completed the intervention. We don't want a signed confession; we want an agreement to accept both an evaluation and the treatment recommendations that usually follow from it.

Selecting Team Members

Your second major function in preparing for an intervention is to select team members.

How do you decide whom to include in the intervention? We want those who have firsthand information and observations about the events and concerns that have precipitated the intervention and who are significant to the individual personally or professionally, or both. The intervention team should include:

1. A coordinator
2. A person(s) who's personally significant to the subject and who has firsthand information to present regarding personal and professional behavioral changes
3. A person professionally significant (employer, partner in practice, representative of a state-level peer assistance program, bishop, hospital administrative personnel, medical staff officer) and who has firsthand information to present regarding professional behavioral changes and

professional practice changes
4. A professional who's in successful recovery from chemical dependence and who may also be one of the above

Who Can Be Included

Selecting team members can be a simple process if you know each potential member's ability to meet the following criteria:

1. Should have a purpose in participating (as above) and **know** that intervention is necessary
2. Should understand the purpose of the intervention and agree to support it
3. Should have and express concern for the subject as a person
4. Should demonstrate some insight into his or her own emotional and behavioral responses to stressful situations (similar to those that occur during the intervention)
5. Should be willing to commit himself or herself to an unrestricted amount of time for the intervention itself
6. Should acknowledge that chemical dependence is a primary disease or be willing to accept education by the coordinator

---

Criteria for Selecting or Excluding Team Members

Selection Criteria	*Exclusion Criteria*
*1. Has a purpose in being on the team.	1. Insists things aren't as bad as they seem.
*2. Acknowledges and supports the purpose of the intervention.	2. Is a primary enabler of the subject.
*3. Expresses concern for the subject.	3. Has an adversarial relationship to or is in direct competition with the subject.
4. Has insight into his or her own personal stress responses.	4. Expresses the need to "get him or her to admit" chemical dependence.
*5. Is willing to commit the time needed.	5. Doesn't support treatment recommendations.
6. Acknowledges chemical dependence as a primary disease.	6. Believes "It's their own fault."
	7. Exhibits anger and mood swings likely to lead to loss of control in intervention.

Of course, not all potential candidates for the intervention team will possess all the desired characteristics. However, it's crucial that they meet to some degree the asterisked criteria (1, 2, 3, 5). If they're ambivalent about the need for the intervention, they may falter when confronted by the subject and agree with the subject's delusion that he or she is being misjudged and is just a victim of circumstance. Moreover, persons who aren't committed to the actual goal of the intervention (evaluation and treatment) are easily tempted to compromise and undermine the efforts of the entire team. This sometimes happens even in the best of situations, when all participants are properly screened, prepared, and seem entirely ready for the intervention. It's foolish to take on a known problem before you even begin; you'll have enough to deal with in keeping the boat upright in stormy waters! Many professionals included merely because of their position or status within an organization don't understand that chemical dependence is a disease, because they've had little opportunity to learn about it. Fortunately, many of them are amenable to being taught. A good briefing about what it is, how it progresses, and how the data already gathered fits together with what we know about the disease will help. Also effective in gaining their commitment to action is their conviction that the disease will get worse and may well prove fatal if not treated. When all else fails, realizing the inevitability and truly serious nature of the illness can mobilize even the most reluctant into action.

Be aware that most of the people you'll need for the intervention have never done one before. They're not sure what may be expected of them, what intervention will be like, or how it will turn out. Their doubts, fears, and reluctance may well surface during your selection process, but that's normal, so don't let it dissuade you from using such people. Even those who have performed hundreds of interventions still have some anxiety before doing one. Those who can discuss their fears will gain a certain amount of support and reassurance simply because they've expressed them, but don't disregard those who don't. They too are unsure and anxious but aren't comfortable admitting it. The stress of an intervention, with all its implications, real and imagined, can reduce even senior administrators to facial twitching, stuttering, and stammering. All would-be participants must be calmly reassured about the purpose of and necessity for the intervention and the need to avoid delay. Actually, some of the best team members turn out to be those who initially seemed the weakest but who came through wonderfully with constant support and encouragement from the coordinator.

In preparing for an intervention at a large teaching hospital, the chief of service of the department was being prepared to play his part. We (authors) had spent hours with him reviewing documentation, narcotic records, and performance appraisals. Although impressed with the need to intervene, he still struggled with the idea that his man "could actually be stealing drugs," and each time more discrepancies turned up in the records, he became more distressed. However, he was a necessary participant because of his position of authority, so we worked closely with him to give him significant support and direction. His surprise and disbelief about what we were finding in the narcotic records indicated a basic lack of knowledge about chemical dependence and how frequently it occurs in physicians. We educated him at every opportunity and repeatedly emphasized the need for intervention. He verbally agreed with us, but his real message to us was "I still can't believe it."

On the day of the intervention, to calm his anxiety we suggested he write down an outline of the plan so that he would feel more secure in knowing exactly what should come next. He wrote, "Introduce coordinator, the physician already in recovery, and state the reason we're here." Despite the fact that it was all in writing, his anxiety immobilized him. As the intervention began he remained speechless for a few long seconds, then finally did get out the first few lines in a shaky voice. But he couldn't recall the names of the persons to introduce them, so they introduced themselves. This tongue-tied professional was a veteran administrator with years of clinical and administrative expertise; he was merely responding to the stress of the situation. He did recover completely from his initial panic and carried on well during the rest of the intervention, needing only minimal nonverbal cuing and support from the coordinator. The intervention succeeded.

Who Shouldn't Be Selected

When in doubt about whether someone meets the criteria for participation, check these exclusion criteria:

1. Continues to deny and minimize. "Things aren't as bad as you think. You're making too much of this," or "He couldn't have taken those drugs."
2. Has been a primary enabler in the situation, defends own actions, rationalizes and offers excuses.
3. Has had an adversarial relationship with the professional who is subject of the intervention.
4. Expresses a need to "get them to admit to what they've done."
5. Doesn't support the need for specified evaluation; sees only the need for counseling or other help.
6. Expresses the belief that what has happened is subject's own fault.

Sometimes it's simpler to evaluate the prospective team players in relation to these exclusion criteria rather than use the inclusion criteria. It's often easier to exclude those who can't be effective participants and then work with those who are left. Unfortunately, in many interventions with professionals, your choices are limited by organizational structure and policy. Still, be as assertive as you can in choosing the team that will be most effective. If you're forced to include someone you have doubts about, you'll have to work diplomatically with this person to get him or her to understand and accept the purpose of the intervention. To avoid trouble, it's wise to choose people who aren't in direct financial competition with the subject for clients or patients.

One of the great strengths of the intervention process is that it's done only to get a sick person into treatment, not from any hope of personal profit for those who carry it out. Their satisfactions come only from helping to restore a colleague to health and full functioning, not from getting rid of a competitor or harassing someone who's merely disliked. Team members should be free of both real and apparent conflicts of interest. For instance, it's wise not to select intervenors who are employed by or who manage treatment facilities to which the subject might be referred unless the subject is perfectly free to choose from among several equally acceptable treatment centers, lest there be coercion, no matter how subtle, to use the intervenor's own facility. Since we really are sometimes forcing people into treatment that initially they neither want nor feel they need, we must make sure we can establish that what we're doing is for their benefit.

Professional intervenors are obviously paid by someone, sometimes by you on a one-case-at-a-time, services-rendered basis, sometimes on salary by a professional association, sometimes by a treatment center. If a treatment center is paying them, the center may well hope for the referral. But you as coordinator must spell out in advance that such connections absolutely won't tilt the choice toward that center. Remember, you're in control of the intervention.

A nursing director in a 250-bed hospital had a staff nurse who needed intervention. The director collected the usual behavioral and record review data and was prepared to proceed, with the assistance of a local peer assistance program. The director and the nursing supervisor were genuinely concerned about the nurse and were, by our selection criteria, excellent team prospects. A recovered nurse from the community was also willing to participate, so the team was formed. However, during team preparation the hospital administrator expressed his disapproval of doing the intervention and clearly preferred just to terminate the nurse: "We shouldn't tolerate this in the hospital." After private discussion with the Director of Nursing, he agreed to let the intervention take place as planned. He arrived uninvited just before it started and said, "I want to see how you're going to get her to admit this." There was no way to dissuade him. He walked into the office (the intervention area) and sat down in a chair that had been strategically placed in preparation for the intervention. Since there was obviously no way to get him to leave, the coordinator calmly but firmly explained the need for control of the environment during the intervention: "... and that includes seating arrangements." The administrator was asked politely to take a seat at the other side of the room and not to speak during the intervention. He reluctantly agreed and took a seat near the door, which would be out of the nurse's direct line of vision. He didn't utter a sound during the intervention, and when it was over and the nurse was being escorted to the treatment facility he asked, "Just what happened here? I must have missed something. She never admitted a thing, but she's gone off to an evaluation!"

When other interventions occurred in that hospital (there were two more that year), he never again asked to sit in.

This administrator was clearly not a member of this intervention, and yet through careful planning and preparation the actual intervention succeeded in getting the nurse to agree to evaluation. Since he kept silent, his presence might even have helped, but it's no mystery why we preferred not to have him as a team member. He wasn't convinced that we could successfully intervene without actual proof of alcohol/other drug use, and he could easily have sidetracked the thrust toward evaluation into a pointless power struggle aimed at extracting a confession.

Preparing Team Members

Preparing team members is your third function as coordinator. Your first step in that preparation is to see to their education about the intervention.

Education

Regardless of how sophisticated your team members may seem in their knowledge of chemical dependence, never assume they're prepared to intervene with someone they know and like, someone they work with, and, most telling of all, someone very much like themselves. So you must allow time to educate the team about how difficult it is to see the disease in someone close. This can't remove the pitfalls, but it will at least warn potential team members about them. It relieves some of their discomfort at not having recognized the chemical dependence and not having acted sooner. Colleagues and friends have difficulty in not feeling guilty for their prior inaction and ignorance, no matter how understandable. To remember that we're dealing with a group of professional caretakers who have missed what was happening to one of their own, and right under their noses, helps us to understand their situation and to say the right words to them now.

Another part of the education needed is to stress the impact that someone's chemical dependence can have on others. This is a good point to make early in the education process; it's easy to agree on and is less threatening to consider than the possible disruption of the team members' personal relationship with the subject or their lingering disbelief that a colleague and friend might really be chemically dependent. It's also easy to use the data you've all collected to stress the inherent risks to your colleague (such as liability suits) if these practice-related problems are ignored. Once team members clearly understand the clinical and legal implications of the alcohol/other drug-use-related symptoms they've observed, they'll more readily understand and more confidently accept the need for intervening.

Team members, particularly those of the same discipline, have trouble facing potential disbarment, loss of licensure, or other board actions invoked when a professional is identified as chemically dependent. We've already mentioned the negative attitude of some professionals toward these punitive actions and toward the authorities that administer them, and at this point we may sense an attitudinal digging in of the heels. Team members need an opportunity to express their concerns and opinions and then be given the facts about the purpose and likelihood of licensure or similar actions in your state. Erroneous opinions and attitudes based on misperceptions should be dispelled. Sometimes the concerns unfortunately are quite real, yet there may be no alternative to eventual board action. In that case your task is to convince the team that inaction is even worse because of the continuing risk both to clients or patients and to the professional involved. It may be impossible to keep the secret. We (authors) have both talked to far too many widows, listened to the anguish of an attorney who never intended to steal from a client's trust fund (much less be discovered), and heard of the suicide of a professional who might have been helped had colleagues lived in reality instead of in a land of wishful thinking where ignoring a problem would somehow magically solve it. Other professionals have focused on avoiding scandal and protecting a colleague from discovery, only to find that their friend has quite literally been protected to death. Professionals who become clean and sober, able to reason again and to work, usually become quite capable of pleading their own cases and eventually regaining license, health, and reputation.

The biggest mistake is to do nothing. One must be firm, sometimes even very tough, in order to be truly kind.

Very few professionals understand that a licensing board's fundamental task is to protect the consumer. We've often assumed that the boards were or should be there primarily for us! To some degree they are, but not to the extent we believe them to be. As governmental appointees, board members serve commissioners and governors who wish at all costs to avoid the injuries, the scandal, and the embarrassment of letting an impaired professional continue to practice or return to practice too soon. They're rarely criticized in the press for taking away a license too hastily or withholding it too long in the name of public safety. On the other hand, if they're too harsh with an individual, only a few people will protest.

Also, expect different levels of program development in each state and in each profession within a state. There may have been quite recent changes in law and procedures, so what you were told was the case may no longer be true. You should check out any such changes and explain them to the team.

For those team members who are closest to the subject personally and who resent the very thought that the problem is chemical dependence, it's helpful to stress the progressive nature of the disease, particularly if one can illustrate by pointing out some known symptoms. Typical team members are reluctant to cause pain to anyone, so pointing out the reality of observable signs of a sickness, not of moral laxity, is often very effective. When a key team participant still expresses ambivalence, bluntness may be needed. If we don't intervene, this person may hurt someone else and very possibly die from this disease. Don't be afraid to be persuasive; the reality of the situation is almost impossible to overstate. "Caring as much about her as you do, are you willing to take the risk of just letting this go on and then having to live with the consequences?" Even with the most hesitant team members this approach has been effective. They still may not totally believe in the probable diagnosis of chemical dependence, but they'll be galvanized into active participation on the intervention team.

Confidentiality

The coordinator must also relay to team members the importance of ensuring confidentiality at all costs. This need for confidentiality begins at the first consideration of intervention and continues throughout the recovery phase. It's a real challenge that will vary in degree of difficulty in various situations. Some team members find it hard to talk about the colleague's problem at all, even with the rest of the team. Others may be caught up in a kind of dubious excitement because something dramatic is about to happen, and they're in on it. You already know how most of us, including professionals, tend to gossip; never mind what we pretend. We're used to saying things to other professionals about clients that of course we wouldn't mention to laypersons, but gossiping about intervention is to be frowned on. Tell your team members to put themselves in their fellow professional's shoes.

There are many ways to ensure confidentiality while you and team members are collecting the data: "I'm doing a chart review of X patients with X diagnosis," "I've begun random checks of all narcotic sign-out sheets," "We're looking at doctors' orders in our next Quality Assurance meeting." We can manage the actual task creatively while affording maximum anonymity. You can help the key team members devise ways that work without starting rumors. When you start collecting data in written form, all team members should give their documentation to one assigned person who will secure the files in a locked area where only that person has access to the records.

This same protocol is followed for copying information from patients' records. Only one team member should do the copying, in privacy, and shouldn't delegate the work to a secretary, tempting as that is. Unfortunately, no matter how discreetly you go about collecting data, people know something is going on, simply because questions are being asked and records are being reviewed. It's bound to look unusual for a Director of Nursing or Chief of Medicine to appear on a nursing unit if this usually happens only on special occasions such as when hospital accreditation teams visit. It also looks unusual to see the head nurse or assistant head nurse together poring over the narcotic books for hours while carefully checking them against patient charts, or locked in the office for hours. Hospital personnel and other professionals are frequently hyperalert and notice the slightest deviation from what's normal (except, of course, signs and symptoms of chemical dependence in their colleagues). Perhaps this hyperalertness reflects a state of heightened awareness useful in detecting an emergency early and being ready to respond to whatever is about to happen. Regardless, expect them to notice everything. So if you as the intervention coordinator are an "outsider" to the setting in which the subject works, don't do the data collection yourself; it will be hard enough for the people who work there regularly to manage the job discreetly.

A hospital administrator in one community used to say, "We knew there was trouble whenever two women (intervenors) appeared wearing suits and carrying briefcases." If you're an outsider, perhaps even known for your intervention work, try to be discreet in your visits to the facility. Peer assistance professionals do develop a reputation within their communities, no matter how self-effacing they are, because they have one line of business soon known to all. The stigma attached to chemical dependence can also be felt by those who are forced to deal with the dependence. No hospital, clinic, or agency wants one of its own to be under attack, much less to be disciplined. The appearance of outside intervenors can look ominous even when they're only paying a social visit to a facility, just as a visit by an FBI man or a narcotics agent would.

The best method of keeping data collecting less obvious is to ask the team member who normally spends the most time in the area where the professional works to discreetly collect the chart information and bring it to an office or a conference room where the team can go over it privately. In the same spirit, we don't want to alert the pharmacy to a particular person when we request narcotic records. We can explain that we're doing an audit of amounts of floor stock required or are doing quality review on medication administration or randomly checking charts against sign-outs.

In preparing to intervene on a nurse who was suspected of diverting large amounts of Fentanyl (a synthetic narcotic), the head nurse requested pharmacy records. The pharmacist was suspicious about why they needed all the Fentanyl records from that particular floor for the past two months and made a comment to that effect to the head nurse. She innocently replied, "We're investigating a diversion problem." She didn't name the nurse, but she didn't have to. The pharmacist was dating the suspected nurse, and he alerted her to the investigation. She called in sick for a week, avoiding confrontation and building a defense for her case. This prolonged the inevitable and risked having the nurse commit suicide or resigning and going to work at another hospital if she felt threatened enough.

Preparing the Team Psychologically

Unlike medical procedures, which use sophisticated equipment, medications, and instruments, intervention is a process whose tools are human beings. However, the same methodical preparation that precedes every successful surgery takes place before an effective intervention. The major difference is that we're preparing people, not laying out instruments. Intervention is obviously most effective when the team is well rehearsed. Think of how athletes train—the long hours and the need for concentration and mental discipline. Athletes mentally focus on the goal, avoid negative thoughts, and try to think of themselves as winners. Like athletes, we must prepare ourselves for intervention and assist team members with their psychological preparation. This involves several actions:

1. Explore feelings and attitudes about chemical dependence in general.

2. Explore how emotionally vulnerable we are to this person.
3. Explore our own defense mechanisms (denial, projection, minimizing, justifying, blaming).
4. Explore how we react when facing tears or hostility.
5. Explore our personal weaknesses that if attacked could leave us vulnerable.
6. Explore our own needs for support systems.

In exploring our attitudes about alcohol/other drug use, we often become aware of how they developed. Many of us have chemical dependents somewhere in our families, so we've developed certain reactions and opinions—usually negative ones—about their behavior. We may have experienced this disease firsthand, but we need to identify those feelings and their origin in order to separate them from the task at hand. Old hurts and old resentments, as well as old habits of defending and rescuing, may still be near the surface.

We need to look honestly at our own use of alcohol/other drugs. In our culture most people drink, and many of us have experience with drugs. We may have been drinking buddies or even used other drugs with the subject of this intervention. It's not uncommon at this stage of preparing for intervention that team members suddenly become aware of their own vulnerability to chemical dependence and express this either verbally or nonverbally by attempting to distance themselves emotionally from other team members and the coordinator as they begin to feel guilty or threatened.

The subject of an intervention quickly detects our negative attitudes. Our words may speak of loving concern, but our feelings may be those of dislike. Much of our communication is nonverbal, so team members need to know what their attitudes are before someone else discovers them. Team members who can't come to terms with their feelings and attitudes, who remain stubbornly angry and hostile, should be replaced. Much better that they admit their feelings and attitudes and bow out than to squelch them by command decision and assume they're gone.

It's also common for team members to be dealing with a drinking/other drug problem at home, in either a spouse or a child, and this intensive inventory and attention to chemical dependence may precipitate a flood of emotions. This may be the first time they've come to grips with what the problem, a problem of their own, **actually** is. They may or may not be able to express this to the intervention coordinator. They needn't be automatically disqualified unless you feel that the intervention process would be too painful for them or unless they appear too unstable to meet the strenuous psychological demands of the intervention. (Some, in fact, have learned enough from training to intervene with a colleague that they've arranged successful interventions for members of their own families.) It's difficult to separate one's emotions from a situation and still react in a spontaneous, caring manner if much of one's energy is tied up in trying to block out those emotions.

Another word of caution: Since intervention can be a very intense emotional experience for a group, team members may transfer to the subject of the intervention the attitudes and feelings they have toward someone in their own lives who is or was chemically dependent. (This phenomenon, called projection, is well known in psychotherapy.) Projection may be evident in a wide variety of nonverbal gestures and postures or in tone and expression when members present data. If this occurs, not all is lost, but you must take control immediately and redirect the flow of the intervention. Strong coordinators will have little difficulty in gently but firmly interrupting a team member and asking the next person to present. The time to explain all this is at the end of the intervention. When people are projecting certain attitudes and feelings toward a chemically dependent professional, they're not consciously aware of where those attitudes and feelings are coming from. But in retrospect they can often identify their feelings as very similar to what they've felt for a significant person in their lives who also is chemically dependent. These team members should have the opportunity of talking this out (see next chapter) and perhaps later even be referred for some help for themselves. The intervention coordinator mustn't forget the goal of the intervention, however, while helping team members process their personal reactions.

In preparing ourselves emotionally, one of the more difficult aspects is to determine how vulnerable we are to the one we're intervening with. If this is someone with whom we've worked for some time, we have a relationship. We've often recreated together, been under fire together, traded a host of confidences and favors. We also maintain an image of this person as having certain traits and qualities, most of them positive. We may admire and emulate such persons and feel a certain bond with them. If so, we need to examine honestly our emotional vulnerability as we sit across from them and present them with information they will at first see as damaging. How will you feel when they accuse you of betrayal or look at you as if to say, "How could you, of all people, do this to me? I thought you were my friend." Understand that the subject will at the time see everyone present, you included, as an enemy, no matter what your relationship has been. Expect it.

This overt rejection can be devastating if we don't arm ourselves psychologically against it. In preparing for this type of confrontation, it's helpful to identify in your mind and on paper exactly why the intervention is taking place and what the facts of the situation are. This will help to restore your perspective and to prepare your emotional defense. Face the fact that for a time you won't be popular with that person, but realize that ultimately he or she may well thank you for what you've done. Just don't expect it on intervention day.

Personal Defense Mechanisms

When we experience mild-to-moderate anxiety we naturally try to reduce it in various ways, especially when we feel personally attacked or threatened. For most of us, the defense mechanisms help us through difficult situations and cause few problems. However, when we're presented with a crisis or painful situation we may use these defenses to such a degree that our perception of reality can become distorted. We've already discussed how the chemically dependent person uses defenses as the disease progresses, but we too are human and should evaluate our own defenses. Here's a brief description of them.

1. **Denial**: refusing to recognize or accept troublesome or painful realities
2. **Rationalizing:** inventing excuses so as to make unacceptable behavior seem acceptable
3. **Blaming:** trying to make other people, places, events, or things responsible for what we or someone else has done
4. **Minimizing:** trying to make something seem less serious than it is
5. **Intellectualizing:** trying to make an unreasonable thing seem reasonable by explaining it away
6. **Justifying:** trying to make right a thing that's dead wrong

Evaluating our habitual defense mechanisms really means examining our usual ways of dealing with unpleasant situations. Do you tend to deny that they exist (blind-man's buff)? Do you ever blame someone else when things don't work out (dumping)? Do you often decide first about a situation and then find reasons to support it (rationalizing)?

We all have patterns of emotional functioning that use at least some of these defense mechanisms frequently, but we don't use all of them all the time. Through feedback from others we may already know our style of dealing with things and whether we deny, rationalize, blame, minimize, intellectualize, or justify. It's crucial that we know our own patterns so that we can predict our reactions under stress. How do you react if you feel under attack or think someone dislikes you? What style of defense do you use when backed into a corner? What if someone attacks your credibility? Do you cry and look helpless? Admit to something that shocks you but without showing remorse? Refuse to admit to anything and seem unable to hear the facts? Shout and threaten to sue? Plead and make promises?

These situations arise in professional interventions, and we must be prepared to maintain our balance despite repeated attempts by the subject to disrupt the flow of the intervention by harassing or dividing the team members. Remember, we're dealing with persons who because of their disease have little ego integrity left. They're feeling attacked and are struggling to survive. They may lash out, make unfair, hostile accusations, misinterpret our motives, lie, blame, and threaten. We must examine our own shortcomings and defenses ahead of time so that we're not lured into battle or into defensive rebuttals, or tricked into pursuing side issues by someone who has very few real weapons.

In this process of psychological preparation it's important to take care of your own well-being and use your own support systems. Many of us use our close friends as sounding boards, share our fears and anxieties with them, and feel accepted despite our uncertainties. For reasons of confidentiality, we won't be able to tell everything we know and are feeling right now, but for most of us as professional helpers and listeners, this is a familiar old problem. We're probably adept at sharing what's upsetting us without identifying anyone. Intervention coordinators or team members who participate in 12 Step programs may do well to attend more meetings than usual while preparing to intervene and immediately afterward. Some people say that spiritual support from others or private prayer and meditation enable them to feel more at ease with themselves, more sure of their motives, and more comfortable with the actual process of intervention, and they consciously build a reservoir of inner peace by setting aside time for these things.

Developing an Action Plan

Developing an action plan is your fourth great function as coordinator—after collecting the data, selecting the team members, and then preparing them for the intervention. An action plan provides in detail the necessary structure for the team to follow during the actual intervention. Its components include: 1) determining the leverage to be used; 2) deciding when, where, and how the intervention will take place; 3) checking insurance coverage for chemical dependence treatment; 4) investigating resources for evaluation/treatment referral; 5) making transportation arrangements; 6) anticipating excuses, and 7) taking safety precautions during and after the intervention. It spells out the who, what, when, where, and how of intervention. All elements should be in place to ensure a tight system with no loose ends or loopholes.

Developing an Action Plan

1. Determine leverage.
2. Decide when, where, and how of intervention.
3. Check insurance coverage.
4. Determine evaluation/treatment referral resources.
5. Plan transportation.
6. Anticipate excuses.
7. Observe safety precautions.

Determining What Leverage Can Be Used

In the context of doing an intervention, leverage means the power we have over an impaired professional because he or she perceives the threat of losing something valuable. Depending on what the profession is, the thing of value might be retaining one's license, continuing as a partner in a firm, retaining a position in a family agency, or being allowed to continue administering the sacraments or teaching a class. The threat of losing licensure is usually the most powerful leverage of all, since loss of licensure threatens not only one's present position but one's ability to continue practicing the profession anywhere.

When we speak of using the leverage available when a professional's license is at stake, we're of course not speaking of bullying anyone but simply of stating the facts about licensure standards in a given state. States differ in the particulars of their requirements for each profession, but we're assuming that what you've documented is unacceptable behavior for a licensed professional, and that's your leverage. In the intervention you'll be making explicit just what's at stake. Know the facts in advance so you'll be sure what that really is.

The professional practice acts define the violations for which there will be disciplinary action. The practice acts are all similar, at least in the medical professions, regarding diversion of controlled drugs, unprofessional conduct, and negligence. State bar associations also have much in common. The range of disciplinary action—probation, suspension, revocation— may depend on the offense and the particular board involved. Remember that though it may be hard to prove that someone's thinking was clouded, the mere purchase of illicit drugs usually involves consorting with known criminals—poor form indeed for an attorney or other professional. Some professional organizations, particularly for social workers and psychologists, take very seriously any charges of sexual acting out with patients yet may prove quite inept in addressing alcohol/other drug dependence.

The precise focus of your leverage and how you'll use it will depend on the subject's current licensure status, the actual need for the license, and the responsiveness of colleagues in that profession if alerted to a colleague's alcohol/other drug use in this situation. There's little point in saying one will report to a regulatory body that can't or won't regulate. Know about available peer assistance or board-level programs for members of the particular profession.

A cardinal rule for any intervention, whether colleague or family intervention, is **never** to make any threat that you're not entirely able, willing, and determined to carry out. It's not enough that you and a few colleagues are willing to follow through. Any organization on which you're relying to do its part of the job if you should fail should actually do it. It's much better to determine this in advance than to find out later that you've gone into battle with a gun that shoots only blanks.

To assess what leverage you have, study carefully the state board's criteria for admitting an impaired professional to rehabilitation (regulatory) programs that are far less severe than the full disciplinary process. Some states don't permit a person who has once been disciplined for chemical dependence to enter such programs; he or she must face the disciplinary board. But many states offer first-time offenders voluntary admission to their rehabilitation program for a two-year-minimum period that usually requires treatment, aftercare, monitoring, documented recovery plans, and strict requirements for reporting any noncompliance.

These rehabilitation programs give wonderful leverage if they're offered during the intervention process, since if the professional enters the program there will be neither a formal investigation nor the embarrassment or humiliation of board hearings. Professionals usually agree to participate in these programs when their only alternative is to walk out of the intervention and take their chances on being reported.

In some states that have programs under the division of licensing and regulation, the statutes require "voluntary suspension" of licensure when a chemically dependent professional is identified; but if adequate treatment, aftercare, and an active recovery plan are arranged and followed and if this is well documented, reinstatement can often follow quickly. These voluntary suspensions are much less damaging professionally than is the ordeal of going through the full disciplinary process—a nasty business at best, even when one is innocent. Again, it pays to learn about the system within which the particular professional works, since rules vary so much. In New York, for instance, the option of voluntary surrender isn't available if a patient has been harmed.

The point is that no matter what programs are in place, maintaining licensure is very important to the subject. Know that and use it to your mutual advantage. Know too that if the state takes the initiative and proves that someone is chemically dependent, there will be no hope of maintaining or regaining licensure without documented chemical dependence treatment. The state will be much more lenient, though, if a professional honestly seeks help rather than being discovered while trying to conceal chemical dependence.

Deciding When to Intervene

The timing of the intervention will be different in each situation. If there seems to be no immediate danger to the subject or to others, a brief delay that enables the group to act more effectively is obviously much better than rushing in precipitously. We like to have at least 24 hours to prepare, much longer if possible. To do all the things we've been suggesting takes time. In some cases, you may have the luxury of ample time if you feel there's little risk in permitting what is probably a long-standing situation to continue a few days more. These are judgment calls you must make in view of the particular situation presented. Have you been able to find out what you need to know about the law? Is a partner who should be part of what you're doing out of town? Is it Friday? Have you had time to finish what you're reading right now? Use your common sense to decide whether you really need or can afford more time or whether you're just procrastinating.

Handling Crisis Situations

Few situations require immediate intervention. Cases like those of a doctor or nurse who was obviously intoxicated while practicing professionally, or of a judge who literally fell off the bench shortly after a liquid lunch, are rather rare but do happen. When they do, the **when** of the intervention is always **now**, and the entire preparation process must be put into high gear. Remember, you may not complete the entire intervention immediately. People can be sent home to sober up and then meet with the team a few days later.

If you're called in as an outside experienced intervenor at a moment of crisis, take a few preparatory steps. Ask whoever called for assistance to start collecting data and to prepare written documentation of what precipitated the crisis. If emergency action has already been taken, usually because someone is intoxicated or has overdosed while on duty, attempt to get blood alcohol level or drug screens if possible. Try to get at least two other discreet people to the scene to observe the subject and testify later as to his or her condition. If the person is working at a hospital, alert the hospital to keep the person on the premises. This can usually be managed by having someone ask the person to stop by the office in an hour to clarify something—or by using any similar delaying tactic. By the time you arrive, there should be enough data to begin.

Team members must be selected quickly. You'll need brief interviews with several persons. Simply select those you feel would handle the situation best. You may need to give them some basic information about chemical dependence (Chapters 1 and 2 will be helpful) and about how important it is to help the colleague and those whose lives are closely intertwined with his or hers.

Actually, in such a crisis you're doing everything at once: reviewing data, selecting and educating team members. If necessary, this preparation process can be completed in 15 minutes. It's been done, believe it or not!

At the end of the intervention, instruct the team to continue assessing data and working until all the key elements have been investigated. This material will be needed if the board requires documentation and if you need to perform a second intervention while the person is on the job or in treatment. People who are admitted to treatment centers are sometimes still intoxicated and confused, and soon after the detoxification period they contest their need to be in treatment. At that point, their denial can easily reestablish itself, so the treatment facility may want help from those who know specifically what events initiated the primary intervention.

These second interventions are usually performed in the treatment center, often with the intervenor, a key team member from the first intervention, and the treatment counselor participating. The data is presented again to the subject, often now greatly expanded, and the treatment team presents treatment observations and recommendations. These second rounds are often very effective for getting professionals to accept treatment and cooperate with it.

A nursing supervisor called for assistance from a nurse intervenor during the early evening hours. She stated that a nurse in the Intensive Care Unit (ICU) had apparently used Demerol and was nodding off in the lounge. Also, the records indicated that within a two-hour period she had signed out 200 mg of Demerol for patients for whom it hadn't been ordered. Since it would take half an hour for the intervenor to arrive at the hospital, the supervisor was requested to 1) have the assistant head nurse in the ICU monitor the nurse closely and offer to do any needed patient-care procedures for her, should she become more alert and attempt to do them herself, 2) copy the narcotic records for the past week, and 3) call the nursing director, inform her of the situation, and ask her please to come to the unit.

By the time the intervenor arrived these tasks had been completed, and the narcotic records clearly indicated that significant dosages of Demerol had been signed out by the nurse in the preceding three hours but that no patient orders on the charts called for Demerol. The assistant head nurse, a close friend of the nurse in question, was present and said she had been concerned about her friend's recent withdrawal, mood swings, forgetfulness, and weight loss. On one previous occasion, at the end of a break a staff member had gone to the lounge to call the nurse back to the unit but couldn't awaken her. This other episode was well documented by the supervisor, and it was decided that although the assistant head nurse was involved emotionally, she could attend the intervention as an advocate for the nurse. The supervisor agreed to present the data, and the Director of Nursing would represent the employer. The intervention was completed only 20 minutes after the nurse intervenor arrived. The nurse was escorted to a treatment facility for evaluation. In this case, the nurse was ready for help and accepted the recommendations without protest.

When the need for intervention is less urgent and the evidence less compelling, there will be time to collect the data methodically, interview the prospective participants, educate the team, write the scripts, and do some role play. There's also more time for exploring the subject's domestic and professional responsibilities, treatment options, and insurance coverage and to plan how to get the person to come to the designated intervention site. Since a chemically dependent professional can easily damage himself or herself (for example, in an automobile accident) and clients or patients as well (for example, by giving wrong legal advice or writing a wrong prescription or botching surgery), don't put off the intervention for longer than a very few days. Remember, once symptoms appear in the workplace, the disease is usually quite advanced and the next crisis unpredictable. Family interventions may be planned for weeks, sometimes months, but a chemically dependent professional may cause harm to self or others at any time. Choose a time of day to fit the situation and the setting. If possible it should be at a time when the person is unlikely to be significantly intoxicated or high, since such a person is rarely capable of sound judgment, especially in the highly charged atmosphere of an intervention.

When dealing with nurses, we prefer to intervene just before they go on duty or just after they come off duty, depending on the information we've received. Of course, if the former, you must arrange coverage for this person who will unexpectedly not be present to cover the assigned shift. By planning the intervention during the normal work routine you can be reasonably sure of catching up with the subject. You need to decide precisely at what time and where to do it in view of the type of professional practice pattern. The place should be available, private, and generally suitable for your purpose (for details, see below). If the subject is somehow forewarned of the intervention, you may have to catch up with the person at some unlikely time or place: during office hours, at the country club, just after a church service, at home, particularly during evening hours. (Even if subjects suspect something's going on, they're less likely to anticipate facing the intervention team during off hours.)

Have the team arrive an hour before the subject does. The team will need that time to prepare, and you need buffer time in case of unexpected minor emergencies such as flat tires, dead batteries, a sick child. Human efforts like these are subject to Murphy's Law: If something can go wrong, it probably will—and usually when you're on a deadline, trying to catch a train, bus, or plane, or doing an intervention. The person you're most relying on may be the very one whose dog gets hit by a car or whose favorite daughter calls to say she's about to leave school to run off with a rock star.

Deciding Where to Intervene

Where the intervention takes place depends on where the subject works. For hospital workers, the hospital is ideal, since it has meeting and conference rooms where one can ensure privacy. For professionals working in a church building or office setting, you'll have to evaluate each place. There are many ways to meet in other locations: For instance, a colleague or friend may invite the subject to meet with him or her, ideally in a place where the intervention can take place undisturbed. Remember, the less likely the place is to stir up suspicion, the better. We want to keep the element of surprise, which is a real asset in an intervention, but we don't want the subject to be frightened and perhaps take impulsive action.

When possible, select a location that will 1) be private, 2) not arouse the suspicion of the subject, 3) comfortably seat all participants without over-crowding, 4) have a telephone in the room for emergency use (for outgoing, not incoming, calls), and 5) provide ample parking spaces so that the cars of team members won't be recognized when the subject arrives. Some of this may sound ridiculous, but we've learned by experience that these factors do enter into ensuring a smooth intervention process. The middle of an intervention isn't the time to be concerned about feeding parking meters or getting to a garage before it closes.

Interventions may have to occur in nontraditional places. For example, a community physician called us to see a nurse who was an inpatient at a local hospital. She worked as a staff nurse at a different hospital in the same city. Her admitting diagnosis was sepsis (a toxic condition caused by pathogenic microorganisms in the bloodstream). When we first saw her she had just been transferred out of Intensive Care and was receiving antibiotics and nutritional supplements. She explained that she had tried some of a neighbor's cocaine and got sick. As we listened to her implausible explanations about her present state and use of cocaine, we began to wonder if she had other drug-use problems at her workplace. At a meeting with her director, the director offhandedly mentioned that Demerol was consistently missing from one of the nursing units—this nurse's unit. Yet when this nurse was away ill, no more Demerol was missing. Moreover, we were told that a recent divorce had caused personality changes in her. Having collected enough data, we conducted an intervention while she was still an inpatient at the hospital. Unfortunately, though, she didn't accept treatment; instead, she was enabled not only by her director (who wouldn't insist that she have an inpatient chemical dependence evaluation after her discharge from the hospital) but also by a mental health professional the nurse had been seeing privately. The nurse returned to work but was later terminated.

This case shows that intervention can take place anywhere if there's sufficient documentation; but it also shows that it can be sabotaged when significant persons engage in enabling—in this case, by refusing to compel the person to at least undergo an evaluation by an expert in chemical dependence. At the time of the initial intervention, this nurse was willing to enroll in the peer assistance program, but in the week that followed she had time to manipulate her co-workers into taking her back with no more than promises of better behavior. Despite attempts by peer assistance to educate the director, she refused to make chemical dependence evaluation a return-to-work condition.

Assessing Insurance and Benefits

Any action plan must include assessment of the subject's health insurance. Many policies don't cover inpatient chemical dependence treatment at all, or do so only minimally. Some will cover treatment in hospitals only; some will include freestanding facilities. Some will cover residential treatment but not pay for outpatient visits or for day or evening programs, even when these are much less expensive and for some chemically dependent people are quite adequate. Average costs of hospital-based inpatient treatment for a 30-day program range from $5,000 to $15,000. This presents a real dilemma when we're recommending a specific very costly treatment to someone who's struggling to survive financially.

Knowing the situation in advance will help you address the issue not only with the treatment center but also with the subject at the time of intervention. Even with additional transportation costs, out-of-state treatment may be less expensive. Since professionals are generally a good financial risk in that they're usually honest and can find work anywhere, anytime, treatment centers will often accept later payments. This can be discussed during treatment. Even when attorneys, priests, nurses, dentists, pharmacists, or physicians have had no financial resources, we've always been able to find a treatment bed somewhere for them.

While checking on insurance protection, also check on other benefits. How much vacation time, sick time, holiday time is available? These benefits will help the patient meet regular ongoing expenses while still in treatment. Check whether private practitioners have disability coverage in addition to hospitalization. Or if recently separated people are still legally married, they're often still covered by a spouse's insurance policy. Angry though estranged husbands and wives may be, they're often willing to help a spouse if it costs them nothing.

Anticipating financial concerns will certainly save time and will help make everyone aware of options at the time of intervention. There are usually many more possibilities than you realize. Experienced social workers are often quite expert at knowing about them, and treatment facilities have an obvious interest in helping patients discover sources of payment.

Securing an Evaluation or Treatment Bed

You must have a definite plan to present to the subject. What actually do you want the person to agree to at the end of the intervention? Whatever you present, expect an attempt to substitute a different plan, such as an offer to see a different person for evaluation—often, of course, a good friend or physician enabler. Subjects will try to accept only part of your plan or try to delay it. Be prepared for this or you may be seduced into compromise, particularly if you're pleasantly surprised by the seeming compliance.

Here are some practical suggestions:

1. If your state has a professional peer assistance program, request a list of treatment centers approved for this professional group. Otherwise, network with other professionals who have had experience in intervention and treatment referrals. Many national professional organizations keep lists of resources and will give information without demanding to know the identity of the person in trouble. (See Appendix H.)

2. Try not to permit treatment centers to recommend themselves; as we've

pointed out, their motives may be mixed. Local not-for-profit agencies such as affiliates of the National Council on Alcoholism are listed in the yellow pages of most large urban areas and usually give relatively unbiased information about competent treatment resources for both alcohol and other drug problems.

You'll soon become aware that there's much discussion of how best to treat fellow professionals. Some say they should ideally be treated with their colleagues and in settings that specialize in treating members of that profession; others say the special treatment they really need is not to be given special treatment. To date, there's no definitive evidence either way. The point of view usually reflects the view of the facility where the advocate of that viewpoint is working or, if the advocate is free of any involvement as a treatment provider, where a personal recovery was achieved.

3. The choice of treatment setting may be based on "I just don't want to be someplace where people know me." This poses no problem, since there are many good places across the country. Or the choice may also be dictated by what's covered by insurance.

4. It's important that for the initial referral and evaluation you select a facility where you can see the subject and where he or she can be admitted at once, preferably that same day. Once the inpatient evaluation is completed, it's possible to transfer a patient (though treatment centers frown on it) to another facility the patient prefers—if it has the expertise to carry out the treatment successfully. Sometimes such a transfer will be arranged by the facility itself if, for example, what seemed initially to be a chemical dependence problem is in fact psychiatric. Some transfers have followed agreement by patient and staff that particular situations such as being positive for the AIDS virus won't be well handled in that setting.

5. Sometimes it turns out that chemical dependents actually do have psychiatric troubles that greatly complicate or even take precedence over their problem with chemical dependence. In such cases, the psychiatric problems may indeed have to be addressed first. But some people whose real problem or major problem is chemical dependence may prefer to be diagnosed as having psychiatric problems and to be referred to a psychiatric facility rather than diagnosed as chemically dependent and referred to a chemical dependence center. Why? First, because they hope to avoid, in their own and others' eyes, the stigma attached to chemical dependence. Second, if their problems are psychiatric, they may be able to continue drinking or using other drugs

(because the psychiatrist may prescribe tranquilizers or antidepressants and may not address the need for abstinence from alcohol /other drugs). Meanwhile, if the psychiatric staff go searching for what they think is the "real cause" of the chemical dependence, the focus will remain on the why of the chemical dependence rather than on the how of recovery—and the subject can go right on drinking or using.

Unfortunately, those psychiatrists who have little understanding of chemical dependence often see chemical dependence as merely a **symptom** of underlying psychiatric problems instead of as a **primary disease** that's often the **cause** of such problems and that therefore should be addressed first to see if the psychiatric problems will dissipate after the person has received treatment for chemical dependence.

Clearly, what we want is a psychiatrist who also thoroughly understands chemical dependence and the complexity of dual diagnosis. Many such psychiatrists who diagnose the subject as having both kinds of problems will prefer to handle the problem of chemical dependence first.

6. A free choice among three or four equally good facilities makes good sense; the freedom to choose one that won't be effective doesn't. Anonymity is a genuine concern, but don't let subjects go treatment shopping. Their illness can make them quite manipulative and crafty, and since they don't yet really believe they need help, their resistance appears in the form of controlling where they'll agree to go. It's ideal to have three equally good places to suggest at the time of intervention, together with the certainty that a bed is available at each of them. Make the selection without delay at the time of intervention. One of these could be out-of-state or at least away from the local area.

7. For women, it's also a good idea to have available a good facility that specializes in the treatment of women. One of us (authors) is firmly convinced that one's identity as a woman is much more important than whatever professional education or work experience one has had and that, whenever possible, treatment in an all-women's place or in a separate women's unit in a larger facility is much more desirable than to be sent to a program designed by and for men. In the latter, the treatment itself will likely be directed by men, and most of one's fellow patients will be men, even if the men are members of one's own profession.

In view of our own experience, we don't believe that there's any one right kind of treatment or center for everyone. Age, drug of choice, ethnic group, sexual orientation, financial resources, presence of other medical or psychiatric conditions (particularly chronic pain problems), availablily to family who may need to be included in the treatment process—all will influence choice. Treatment selection is a highly individualized affair, and very different approaches should be offered to different persons. You don't need to know all about these places, but it's good to have input from people who are familiar with a variety of good possibilities and who have no vested interest in recommending one over another.

Arranging for Transportation

Since we're planning to intervene with someone who can't meet standards of practice and whose behavioral unpredictability we've carefully documented, it isn't wise to allow the person to drive himself or herself either home or to treatment. Such persons may still be under the influence of alcohol/other drugs or in early withdrawal and will certainly be preoccupied and upset. Some may even be contemplating suicide. Many recovering healthcare professionals say that the thought of suicide was strongest immediately after intervention and before they had any opportunity to believe in recovery or feel any realistic optimism about the future. It seems reasonable for subjects to want to go home, pack some clothes, and tend to a few details, but those details may involve telling a none-too-supportive spouse what has occurred and announcing unexpectedly that they're about to leave for a month. Not an easy task at best! Remember, too, that many people have never seen a specialized treatment center and don't anticipate a warm, friendly, nonjudgmental setting. If their only experience has been with mental hospitals or watching movies like "Lost Weekend," they may be feeling real terror. This is where another experienced professional in recovery may be able to reassure them and give them some idea of what to expect. It's also helpful at this point, if you do know the name of the physician or counselor who will be working with them, to let them know who the person is.

On rare occasions a subject who has been allowed to leave an intervention unescorted while feeling helpless, worthless, and very depressed has committed suicide. This is indeed rare, but it's a possibility, and planning should include ways to prevent it. Arrangements may be made for a colleague, friend, or another professional in recovery to escort the person to the treatment center (or home if something urgent must be taken care of there). If the subject is under the influence of alcohol/other drugs at the time of intervention, it's advisable to have two persons serve as escorts, since the person's perceptions may be distorted, especially in light of the upset precipitated by the intervention, and his or her behavior may be impulsive and unpredictable. Intoxicated people may suddenly become assaultive, may demand a drink and become very unruly, even physically difficult to control, if it's denied them. No one escort should risk having to handle those possibilities while trying to drive a car.

By following the steps of the intervention plan presented in this book, you'll be providing your impaired colleague with structured support, genuine caring, and honest concern—all of which minimize the possibility of physical harm.

Anticipating Excuses from the Professional

The impaired colleague may have legitimate excuses for not wanting to cooperate with the team. What if the subject feels unable to comply with the team's recommendation for treatment because he or she is a single parent, is married but has no full-time babysitter for a young child, has cats or a dog, a parakeet, horses, whatever? These may not seem to be world-shaking problems, but they're real concerns that must be dealt with. Oddly, children are often less of a problem than pets are, because one can often find a family member to take care of children for a month, and some treatment facilities accept both mother and baby. (In some cases, though, we've had to fly children out-of-state to stay with relatives or friends.) If there really is no one to take care of children (and sometimes this is hard to ascertain, since the subject will gladly use them as excuses for "why I can't go"), there may be a network of colleagues or friends willing to give such care. If you've exhausted every other possibility, there are almost always emergency placement services available through local social agencies.

When the subject flatly refuses to enter treatment, child protection services may be consulted, because an impaired parent can harm a child. In some states, the law provides that chronic alcohol/other drug abuse may render one automatically guilty of child abuse. When faced with this information, the subject will frequently remember someone in the family who can care for the children.

Pets can be taken care of in a variety of ways. Neighbors will frequently be willing to feed the bird, cat, or goldfish; dogs can be boarded with friends or family for a month. If not, members of professional support groups will usually come to the rescue. Looking out for children and pets is one more "to do" for anyone who does interventions on a regular basis. Keep a resource list of local professionals and laypeople in recovery who might be willing to help. One person had five children yet offered to do child care for any colleague needing treatment. She said, "When you have five, what's a couple more?"

Taking Safety Precautions

We must realize that in doing an intervention we're creating a crisis for the subject, no matter how necessary it is and no matter how lofty our motives. The outcome may be wonderful, and months from now a grateful colleague may be singing our praises, but today we're disrupting a life. This disruption can seem devastating to one who's already in trouble and struggling to keep things together, even with the "help" of alcohol/other drugs. Most painful of all is our implied but clear message: "You're not capable of helping people anymore," which is interpreted as "You're a failure." Because of their illness and the stress of the situation, chemical dependents are often incapable of processing information normally and will hear what we're **not** saying, no matter how clearly we spell out our positive regard and real concern for them.

People under attack are capable of extreme behavior if they believe it necessary to protect themselves, so they can be violent. If you've observed patients with cocaine-induced psychosis or who have overdosed on amphetamines, you already know the signs of paranoia or delusions of persecution. It's not only the drug that may lead to violence, but also the distortion of reality caused by drug use. There may already have been many losses, and the intervention may be seen as yet one more threat. The intervention may trigger intense emotion that the subjects may have difficulty controlling because they may feel they're losing control of everything.

In view of the dangers of the situation, then, do these things to prepare your safety net:

1. Have a telephone in the room for (outgoing) emergency calls if you should need security assistance or psychiatric help, and know the numbers in advance.
2. Have psychiatric backup readily available should an involuntary admission be needed.
3. Follow seating guidelines indicated in the next chapter.
4. Watch for signs that the subject may be carrying a weapon, and find out if this person has ever been known to carry one.
5. Obtain a description of the make, model, and license number of the subject's car.
6. Have the home and work phone numbers of the spouse or significant other or friend.
7. Have phone number of the professional's private physician.

Remember: It's normal for people who feel cornered to respond at times with fight-or-flight reactions. These reactions are the exception during intervention, but they do occur, so it's well to be prepared for them.

Addressing the "What Ifs"

People preparing an intervention always worry about the "what ifs." "What if he won't agree to evaluation or treatment?" "What if she walks out and won't even listen?" "What if she never talks to me again?" "What if he gets violent?" "What if she sues?" "What if he ends up harming himself?" On and on! All of us who perform interventions still go into every one of them with some such anxieties. Your fifth major function as coordinator is to help the group address these "what ifs."

The questions discussed below are ones we're asked everywhere we go. Some of them refer to serious and even frightening problems, and we answer them as honestly as we can, because they're realities we have to face. At the same time, the answers are ultimately reassuring, because they can give you the confidence that comes when you've thought of all the problems in advance and have prepared a plan that can handle them if they really do come up.

What If They Won't Go to Evaluation?

If they won't go, it can mean several things. They may not believe they have a problem and are maintaining strong denial despite all your attempts to introduce some reality. They may know they have a problem but are fearful of having it disclosed. They may not believe you really will do more than scold and threaten. Or, faced with the reality of losing their drugs, they'd rather sacrifice the job than give them up. So what can you do?

1. Don't give up. Repeat the intervention steps outlined in Part II, several times if necessary, emphasizing the **alternatives** (using your leverage).
2. Since one of your team is a professional who's already in recovery, it can help a great deal if this person talks about the problems he or she has faced and is conquering. This self-disclosure or identification with the subject is most encouraging, since people in deep trouble tend to think no one else has ever faced such problems.
3. If the above steps fail, you must evaluate the dangers that an uncooperative subject might pose to self and/or others, and then consider what can be done. For instance, might the subject be a candidate for involuntary admission to a psychiatric unit to protect him or her from harming self or others?
4. Is there a state statute that provides for involuntary admission to treatment programs for alcoholics or other drug-dependent persons through legal proceedings?
5. Can you get the subject's attention in other ways? For example, do you have other significant data that you hadn't planned to use but now might

117

have to resort to, such as making reports to child-protection services or filing legal or criminal charges? (As we've mentioned, in some states the law provides that chronic alcohol/other drug abuse may render one automatically guilty of child abuse.)

6. If all these attempts don't obtain the desired result, you may have to let go, knowing you've given it your best, and initiate the appropriate procedures. That may include getting the person dismissed from a firm or facility, notifying other employers (of someone who moonlights), reporting to the licensing board or professional association, and in severe cases where client or patient safety is endangered, requesting immediate suspension of the license to practice. This last action is rarely taken and requires cooperation from the attorney general, but it may have to be done.

What If They Walk Out at the Very Beginning?

This situation is difficult in that you've had no opportunity to present the objective data (reality) to the subject. Depending on the circumstances, there are several ways to deal with this:

1. If there's no immediate danger to clients or patients, reschedule the intervention and notify subjects in writing that if they don't come, disciplinary procedures will be promptly initiated by the employer and through the licensing board or other regulatory group. This usually will get their attention, even though it also makes them angry and indignant, and they may attend, if only to "give you a piece of my mind."

2. If subjects appear extremely dangerous, you can initiate a request for immediate licensure suspension through the licensing board, and the employer may also bar them from the premises where they practice. In most cases, to request a "summary suspension" successfully, one must provide the board with detailed and documented evidence of the subject's inability to practice safely. At the same time, if a state statute provides for involuntary admission to treatment for chemically dependent professionals, explore what the legal requirements are and how to initiate proceedings. If there's significant concern about the subject's own safety, a call made to notify the family of what's taking place and to ask their assistance may be in order.

What If They Take Legal Action?

The chance of this happening is minimal. To safeguard against it, though, careful documentation is critical, because it can establish why you took action and can make it clear that the intervention was based on objective practice issues, not on an unjustified personal vendetta or professional jealousy. Remember, you haven't labeled anyone or made a diagnosis. You've simply pointed out unacceptable behavior related to professional practice and insisted only that the person be evaluated and that treatment (if needed) be chosen by an expert on the basis of that evaluation. It's very difficult to dispute objective evidence and carefully gathered documentation.

Many states have "hold harmless" clauses for those who report colleague impairment provided they take action in good faith; other states will hold you liable if you knowingly **fail** to report a dangerous situation.

Here are two suggestions:

1. If you're threatened with legal action, communicate with the attorney relaying the threat. Often the subject has misrepresented the situation, and it's easy to clarify what actually happened. Sometimes one can even enlist the attorney's support in urging evaluation and treatment, particularly if the evidence on which the intervention is based is well documented.

2. If you're named in litigation, don't panic. We know of no successful lawsuits brought against intervenors who have been thorough in their preparation. Most attempted suits are never even taken to court, because the accuser must prove things that hardly ever happen—for instance, that the intervenors profited from their allegedly wrongful accusation, that they invented their data, gossiped, treated the chemically dependent professional brutally or carelessly, or acted as if they were professional diagnosticians. A colleague can hardly claim to have been ill used when intervenors have simply been trying to protect the public from an impaired colleague by getting that colleague into evaluation and treatment rather than letting him or her face the agony and possible disgrace of a disbarment proceeding or revocation of license.

What If They End Up Killing Themselves?

The blunt fact is that any chemically dependent person is a potential suicide, whether deliberately so or by overdose or other kind of accident. Our own experience and major studies of suicide clearly confirm that truth. What we can and must do is take precautions against such a tragedy. Essentially that means that we get such persons into the safe environment of a treatment facility and continue to express our loving concern. Beyond that we can do little in a practical way, because we're dealing with a high-risk group of people, some few of whom do kill themselves even in psychiatric hospitals with suicide precautions in full effect.

Dealing with suicide is an extremely painful experience if we've had even the remotest relationship with the person. We and anyone else associated with the person may be tempted to give in to guilt feelings: "If only I had been there. . ." "If I hadn't said those things. . ." "If only I had alerted her husband. . ."

If, rare though it is, a suicide should occur, we must look realistically at the question of blame. The overall principle is that **we simply can't take responsibility for the subject's action**. To repeat, we're dealing with a high-risk group. We have only two weapons: personal persuasion expressed through loving concern, and the threat to a subject's ability to continue in practice. Sometimes a subject rejects both of these with "Go ahead and take my license. I was going to stop practice anyhow!" (Married women in particular, who may have mixed feelings about trying to combine career and homemaking, may say that sincerely and receive considerable social support if they do.) If at that point the subject can neither be committed nor jailed— even if the intervenors are willing to go to that extreme—intervenors are essentially helpless. Their consolation then consists in knowing that they've honestly done everything they could; the rest is out of their hands.

A young woman veterinarian was referred to a peer assistance program after being admitted to a six-month-long outpatient chemical dependence treatment program. At the time of her admission to the outpatient program (after referral by her employer for suspected diversion of drugs) she was so markedly depressed that she had begun psychiatric counseling sessions as well. The psychiatrist prescribed antidepressants because of her severe mood swings and severe depression. Also during this time she secured new employment at an emergency animal clinic.

On the initial intake performed by the peer assistance program, it was discovered that this subject was taking not only prescribed antidepressants but also various tranquilizers and sedatives. Considering her history of drug diversion and current drug use it was recommended that she have a complete chemical dependence evaluation at an approved facility in order to be enrolled in the peer assistance program. After this evaluation the team recommended intensive outpatient treatment for chemical dependence. She voluntarily enrolled in the program, which also required that she remain free of all mind-altering drugs.

During the following months she remained moody, unpredictable, defensive, and began to talk to close friends about killing herself. These people didn't share this information right away, but when her threats became more frequent they notified the peer assistance program. At the same time her friends called the program, her employer called to say that her job performance was deteriorating, her absenteeism was increasing, and her behavior was suspicious. She often flew into a rage with no provocation, appeared listless and "spaced out," and her speech was often disjointed. A urine screen was performed by the employer while the peer assistance program prepared to intervene, using her friends as team members. The intervention was successful, and she agreed to submit to an inpatient treatment program. The urine screen report received after her admission was positive for several classifications of mind-altering drugs.

While in treatment she apparently didn't face all her problems. She began to distance herself from the peer assistance program and wouldn't sign releases for her counselors to communicate with people working in that program. (It's not unusual for patients to harbor resentment toward those who put them in treatment, but it's unusual that those feelings aren't resolved before discharge.)

She was released at the end of her 28-day program and returned to work without support, guidance, or direction from the peer assistance program. Without releases, the peer assistance program couldn't serve as an advocate for her or as a resource to the employer in preparing for her return to work.

Through other peers in recovery, the peer assistance program became aware that she was enrolled in aftercare at the center and also participating in their professional recovery group.

Within three weeks of her discharge from residential treatment, she was found dead at home from a multiple drug overdose.

This is truly an unfortunate case. Despite several tactical errors, most involving poor communication or the concealment of important information by well-meaning colleagues, this young woman had received support from many sources. She had been exposed to two types of chemical dependence treatment, been offered support by concerned colleagues, seen at least two psychiatrists and had both group and individual therapy, yet ultimately died. Whether her death was intentional or accidental will never be known and perhaps really isn't the issue. Sometimes doing all we can do is simply not enough.

Unexpected and seemingly unncessary death is one of the most painful parts of dealing with chemical dependence, particularly when we've made great efforts to help. The sad record of how many chemically dependent people meet an untimely death can teach us a powerful lesson: **Don't sit around and worry. Act now.**

We've had a number of failures. With what we know now, many probably could have had happy endings, but we did the best we could at the time. We've faced a lot of anger, and our motives have often been questioned. Sometimes after treatment the anger turned to understanding and acceptance, even gratitude. Sometimes treatment never even happened.

We may wish we had been more skillful, but we don't regret any of our attempts to help. What we do regret is not doing anything and thereby losing a colleague. It's hard to admit that a friend was in trouble, suffered permanent brain damage, brought harm or even death to someone else, and that we didn't even care enough to try to help.

Chapter Highlights

Chapter 4 has discussed in detail how the coordinator facilitates early preparations for intervention. The coordinator's chief functions are these:
1. Directs data collection process.
2. Selects team members.
3. Prepares team members.
4. Develops an action plan.
5. Addresses team members' anxieties ("what ifs").

Here are the highlights of each of those functions.

Data collection includes:
1. The precipitating event(s)
2. Evaluation of professional performance and current professional status
3. Assessment of changes in interpersonal relationships
4. Learning of medical signs and symptoms/consequences
5. Evaluation of family/social systems
6. Evaluation of legal data

Criteria for selecting each team member are:
1. Has a purpose in being on the team.
2. Acknowledges and supports the purpose of the intervention.
3. Expresses concern for the subject.
4. Has insight into own personal stress responses.
5. Is willing to commit the time needed.
6. Acknowledges chemical dependence as a primary disease.

Preparing the team includes:
1. Education about chemical dependence
2. Discussion of confidentiality issues

3. Psychological preparation: exploration of attitudes and feelings about chemical dependence
4. Identification of personal defense mechanisms: denial, rationalizing, blaming, minimizing, intellectualizing, justifying

Action plan includes:
1. Determining leverage
2. Deciding when and where to intervene
3. Handling crisis situations
4. Ascertaining insurance coverage and benefits
5. Planning for transportation after intervention
6. Anticipating excuses
7. Initiating safety precautions

Addressing team members' anxieties ("what ifs"):
For this, see pages 117-122.

Chapter 5

Phase One: Final Preparations

After completing the preparation outlined in Chapter 4, you're almost ready for the intervention. At this point you may be somewhat overwhelmed by the seemingly endless details, but it helps if you realize that the intervention itself is really 90% preparation. However, the actual intervention does require careful orchestration and thoughtful use of everything you've prepared, and it can be quite stressful.

There are now several steps to go through to ensure that the team members are prepared for a coordinated presentation: 1) defining for them the roles they're to play (this includes identifying for them three other rather undesirable roles they may be tempted to play, showing them how to be an effective group, and helping them identify ways to express their feelings and their genuine concern for the impaired professional); 2) writing the script; 3) establishing ground rules for the intervention; and 4) rehearsing the intervention on the day it will occur.

Defining Roles for the Team

One of the greatest anxieties for people getting ready to participate in an intervention is uncertainty about what is expected of them. Usually one person will say aloud what the others are thinking: "What exactly do I have to do and say?" Regardless of team members' competence, training, or experience in their professional field, we're placing them in a very unfamiliar and decidedly uncomfortable situation that makes them feel as if they're getting ready to fire someone. For instance, one might expect mental health professionals (psychiatrists, psychologists, clinical nurse specialists) to know already what to do in an intervention, but their background experience is often very different. They may be used to being deliberately rather passive and nondirective while asking questions in such a way that patients themselves arrive at correct decisions, and they're trained to keep their feelings to themselves. But intervenors must tell and show the subject what **others** know, feel, think, and want to have happen. Moreover, a major decision is to be made and implemented within minutes or hours, which isn't at all like the slow, thoughtful pace of most psychotherapy.

In order to reduce anxiety we need to prepare each person individually for the specific role he or she will play during the intervention. For example, in addition to the coordinator's critical role, a typical intervention on a colleague may include these roles:

1. Colleague/Friend

This role is pivotal. (There may be more than one colleague/friend.) This person has not only seen firsthand some of the changes wrought by alcohol/ other drug use, but also has some meaningful relationship with the subject. This relationship of friend and co-worker plays a powerful role in breaking through the defenses of the impaired professional. A colleague is, after all, someone like oneself, one from whom we expect support, not supervision or criticism. The colleague is an equal, not a boss.

2. Supervisor, Chief of Staff, Department Head, or Senior Partner

Such persons represent professional authority because they've had administrative responsibility for the subject's professional performance and have been able to judge and document that professional performance. But they may also have enjoyed a long-term collegial relationship with the impaired professional. If so, each may well have held the other in high personal and professional regard. So such persons can wield significant double leverage.

3. Employer or Chief Administrator

The employer role holds a significant power of presence that clearly defines the serious nature of the intervention, a role very helpful in conveying to the professional how important his or her situation is to the organization. When employers are the only participants with any formal leverage, they present the expectations of the institution and the consequences of noncooperation. To a long-term professional employee this person has even greater authority. When this person lays down the law or promises support, professionals believe what's said. Finally, this person represents an institution where the long-term professional has accrued benefits and privileges and, more importantly, may have achieved a level of professional status that's not easily transferred elsewhere.

4. Peer Assistance Program Representative

In states where there are active peer assistance programs for impaired professionals, their representatives often have experience in intervention and can greatly contribute to the effectiveness of the intervention team. These representatives may have no information about the specific case you're now handling, but in reviewing the data you've gathered they may confirm the need for intervention and also state this to the professional. In interventions where there's no employer, such as in the case of a doctor or attorney in private practice, the peer assistance member may tell the impaired professional the expected outcome of the intervention: that the subject will voluntarily submit to a formal evaluation to determine the cause of the documented problems and to recommend treatment if it's needed. Also, the obvious fact that they're representatives of a formal program precisely for professionals who are having problems shows effectively that other professionals have faced the same kind of problems; they're not alone.

5. Professional in Recovery

Professionals now in recovery play a unique role during intervention: that of advocate. They have no vested interest in presenting any information about the subject's behavior; they're there simply to help. They understand the subject's distress, and they offer support and reassurance. No matter how supportive, caring, and nonthreatening other team members are (and they should constantly exhibit those qualities), the impaired professional often suspects a set-up or senses a personal attack. But a colleague in recovery can and should, at an appropriate time in the intervention, share with the subject his or her own personal experience with chemical dependence. This sharing helps the subject to get rid of the feeling that he or she is the only attorney, priest, doctor, nurse (or whatever the position) who has ever had serious problems with chemical dependence. The self-revealing testimony of the professional in recovery gives the subject a glimpse of hope that there is a way out of his or her problems. Such colleagues, in short, are in a special position of oneness with the subject in knowing and speaking of problems that **we**—people like **you and me**—face.

We must remind you that **the roles just outlined must not be considered as the only ones or as inflexible.** The exact role that team members assume will vary according to who they are, the information they have about their colleague, their relationship with the colleague, and their professional status or role within an organization, social group, institution, or agency. It will also depend on the availability of others to assume certain roles. In some situations one person may wear several hats, but we try to minimize this so that the subject receives a clear message from each participant. In other words, a colleague who is both a friend and a supervisor can effectively combine those roles, because a supervisor will have documentation of the practice problems, and a friend will have genuine concern and caring for the individual. But if we were to ask this person to assume the role of representing the employer, he or she would have great difficulty in switching these roles, and the message to the impaired professional would be confusing. (Is this person a colleague, or a disciplinarian?) The subject may exploit such confusion quite effectively.

Despite your careful planning, people under pressure may take on **certain additional roles** as they revert to behaviors that reduce their own stress. Also keep in mind that your team members, no matter how limited their interactions with one another prior to this experience, are developing into a unified group. They're united to work toward a common goal under very stressful conditions, and this creates a certain bonding, no matter how brief the experience. The individuals undoubtedly develop roles to meet their own needs. Here are three common roles that call for comment.

1. Caretakers

Caretakers are people who try to meet someone else's needs—even everyone else's needs. Their interactions usually enhance the ability of the group to work toward its common goal. The emotional intensity of the task at hand also may create a feeling of interdependence and a kind of foxhole camaraderie. Members will increasingly seek support and reassurance from one another and from the emerging caretaker or caretakers as the moment of intervention approaches.

But even early in the preparation process you may begin to see problems created by caretakers. They may start to take responsibility for tasks already assigned to others and may spend much time and energy offering support and reassurance to all. During the rehearsal, the team players will not only look for direction from the coordinator but will look for support from one another, especially the caretakers among them. After all, caretakers do act as strong nurturing figures who provide constant reassurance and even physical gestures of pats on the shoulder or knee, or an arm around a shoulder.

Caretakers are welcomed especially by members who feel insecure, uncertain, and generally anxious during intervention; they can therefore be quite a stabilizing force. They usually know that they're not to take care of the subject during the intervention. However, their caretaking concerns can easily transform them into enablers (a role to be discussed next). But even if they manage to avoid enabling, they may create another problem: They may need special attention from the coordinator at the end of the intervention process. The reason is that they may have great empathy with the subject and hence experience many of the subject's own feelings but may block those feelings during the intervention as they tell themselves they must be strong and take care of other team members. But when the intervention is over and they can no longer focus on others, their own pent-up emotions may pour out, and they may feel quite vulnerable.

2. Enablers

If caretakers are a mixed blessing on a team, enablers (as well as our third group, persecutors) clearly don't rise even to those heights.

It's natural to assume that someone on the team will exhibit enabling behavior during the intervention. The fact that we choose colleagues who have some relationship with the impaired professional often means that they've already enabled this person and may subtly fall into these patterns during the stress of intervention. These friends don't want to risk rejection or retaliation. When confronted by an angry, hostile, or tearful reaction, they may question the actual need for the intervention and begin to align themselves with the subject. They may lose objectivity and present their script with uncertainty. (We discuss the script in the next section.) When challenged by the impaired professional, they may back down and agree that there are plausible explanations for the documented unacceptable behavior or performance or may allow the subject to present the team with rationalizations for each incident. They may agree with or even provide excuses for the professional's inability to comply with the recommended evaluation despite the extensive preparation of the team in anticipating all possible excuses.

The enablers of course aren't consciously aware of what they're doing, and the coordinator may need to redirect, encourage, and reinforce such people. If the situation becomes detrimental to the flow of the intervention, they may have to be asked to refrain from comments until later. The leader can handle this smoothly by saying, "Peter, thank you for sharing your comments.

We'll come back to you later" or "Let's hear from Mary now." When enablers surface during intervention, both the leader and the group must respond swiftly to maintain momentum and to draw the impaired professional's attention away from the enabler and to other members.

3. Persecutors

Sometimes, as we mentioned earlier in passing, the stress of intervention may prompt a group member to project onto the impaired professional the feelings he or she has had in other experiences with chemically dependent persons. Most often this projection stems from a very personal relationship with a chemically dependent spouse, lover, or family member that has caused the team member significant distress. Such persons unconsciously attribute the same characteristics to the subject and express their anger, disgust, and frustration both verbally and nonverbally. Their tone of voice may be judgmental or condescending so that the subject responds with denial, defensiveness, and hostility. The concerns such team members express sound more like accusations. This kind of unconscious, hostile communication by a team member tells the impaired professional that he or she is being judged not as ill but as culpable and deserving of punishment.

Persecutors may also develop these attitudes because of their outrage that any attorney, clergyperson, doctor, or nurse, with such education and advantages, could stoop so low as to become an addict who steals drugs, or a common alcoholic who comes to work drunk. Many healthcare professionals have great difficulty accepting chemical dependence as a disease; they still believe it's a social or moral problem. Although team members have been informed that it's prevalent in the professions and that it's really a disease, they may still assume a persecutory posture when, with the intervention in full swing, they realize the impact of what's being presented. The few minutes or hours we've been devoting to giving new information simply isn't enough to counteract years of prejudice and antipathy. Ultimately, the role some team members assume is based on their disdain for the subject's supposed moral weaknesses and their fear of damaging their image of the profession they practice.

Persecutors are a challenge to deal with during the actual intervention, since their behavior is motivated by their own needs and feelings rather than by those of the impaired colleague. Even though the group leader usually has anticipated each individual's potential for developing counterproductive roles in the selection process, he or she should be alert to the early signs of role change. Some team members will respond to simple nonverbal cues from the leader to change their posture or eye contact, but others will need the leader to interject or redirect the intervention appropriately.

Understanding that intervention is an interpersonal process should prepare us to expect people to react as people, particularly under conditions of pressure. Despite the presence of caretakers, enablers, and persecutors, the leader who expects, identifies, and addresses them properly can lead the group through a successful intervention.

There may be rare situations where because of the urgency of the case, lack of resources, or immediate need for intervention, you may have only two persons available to intervene. If so, it's most effective for one intervenor to assume the role of friend and colleague and the other to assume a role that includes the care and concern of a colleague but also asserts the leverage and authority of an employer or the equivalent in making clear to the professional that these behaviors are unacceptable practice and that there must be a formal evaluation. An intervention team comprised of only two persons is difficult in that they must handle alone the emotional impact usually shared by a team of four to five. Almost inevitably, one of them becomes the "bad guy." After all, one of the two must say clearly that we expect the subject to submit voluntarily to an evaluation process and to follow the recommendations of the evaluating treatment team "or else." The coordinator should warn that whoever does this inevitably becomes the object of the subject's anger and hostility but should emphasize that this shouldn't be taken personally, because the impaired professional is simply trying to preserve self-esteem in a situation where he or she has no influence or control.

Writing the Script

You as coordinator should develop the actual outline for the script with the participation of team members. Use the simple, time-tested format given here. As the group follows the outline, each team member should write his or her script on a piece of paper and later use it in the rehearsal and in the actual intervention.

Writing the Script

1. Introductions
2. Purpose of meeting
3. Presentation of data
4. Interpretation of data
5. Recommendations and alternatives
6. Support from colleague in recovery
7. Repetition of concerns and data
8. "Bottom line" statement
9. Closure

---

1. Introductions by Coordinator

The coordinator will introduce the team players to the subject, since the subject usually doesn't know one or two of them. It helps to identify those persons by their titles if they represent the professional society's programs, state-level peer assistance programs, or local professional intervention groups. This will immediately establish the serious nature of the meeting and encourage the subject to stay and listen well. When professionals in recovery are present, it's best to introduce them initially by name and not say they're in recovery. This can be disclosed later at an appropriate time.

Some examples of introductory statements are:

1. An intervention with an attorney in private practice; the leader is both a colleague and a friend: "Hello, John. I'd like to introduce you to several people you may not know." (He gestures to each in turn.) "This is Robert Smith from the State Bar Association. This is Harry Jones." (Mr. Jones is a fellow attorney known to the subject; he has been in recovery for many years.) "And of course you need no introduction to Alice and Cynthia." (Alice is the firm's executive secretary; Cynthia, a practice partner.)

2. An intervention with a professional working in a hospital where the leader of the intervention team is the subject's head nurse and direct supervisor: "Mary, here are some people who would like to speak with you for a few minutes." (She gestures to each in turn.) "Mrs. Donaldson; Susan Grant; and of course your friend Sarah and the evening supervisor, Ms. Craig." (Mrs. Donaldson is Director of Nursing; Susan Grant is a person in recovery.)

3. An intervention directed by a state-level program intervenor on an impaired surgeon: "Hello, Dr. Smith." (He offers a handshake.) "I'm Jack Turner from the Massachusetts Medical Society." (He gestures to others in turn.) "And of course you know most of these people except Dr. Randall." (Present also are an anesthesiologist who has worked with Dr. Smith for many years; his scrub nurse; and the Chief of Surgery, who is also a close friend of the subject.)

2. Statement of the Purpose of the Meeting

This statement should be broad in scope and yet specific as to how the area of concern relates to professional practice. The tone should be nonthreatening, because we want to gain some degree of trust from the subject, no matter how slight it is—or at least not total mistrust. Introductory remarks should also express the positive esteem, care, and concern that all the team members and other colleagues feel for the subject. Emphasize that before the observed deterioration in professional practice, colleagues and the employer alike have had great respect for the person.

A typical opening statement, then, might go something like this. "John, we're here to discuss with you some matters that have come to our attention in connection with your professional practice. I'm sure you know how much all of us and all your colleagues as well—respect you as a talented, dedicated lawyer [psychologist, counselor, surgeon, or whatever]. Not only that, but many of us are personal friends of yours, and we like you immensely as a person. So we're here today because we respect you and like you. But it's precisely because of our respect and affection for you that we're so much concerned about you and what's been happening in your professional practice. Frankly, the problems have been piling up lately, as the people here will share with you, and what you've been doing isn't like you at all.

"For instance, your office help [or the nursing staff, or whatever] say you often show up late at the office, forget appointments, are sarcastic with clients [patients]. You recently lost a case that you should have won easily, and it cost your client thousands of dollars [or: you showed up for surgery late and could hardly handle a very routine appendectomy]. All of this indicates a real deterioriation in your professional practice, and it's clearly harming you, the people who work with you and love you, and of course your clients [patients] who are depending on you."

As part of the introductory statement, the coordinator also tells the subject, "We'll ask you to let us present our information to you, and we request that you don't interrupt until we've finished speaking. Then you may ask questions and respond fully to what we've said," or "We're going to ask you to hear us out. Please concentrate on listening, and please don't interrupt until we've finished. You'll have ample time to speak and ask questions then. Will you agree to that?" This must be stated in a caring yet firm way, restating that those present are there because they care and are concerned. It's good to get the subject's agreement to listen, since any attempts to rebut and argue can then be more easily controlled by referring to that agreement.

3. Presentation of Data

Team Member 1: This person usually carries the most weight professionally and, if it's a medical situation, presents objective data with specific dates, times of medication discrepancies, charting discrepancies, errors in judgment, and patient-related problems. In organizational healthcare settings, this is usually the first-line manager or head nurse; or in a peer assistance intervention it may be someone who holds a position with the program. This person's presentation serves two purposes: 1) establishing definitely for the subject what the meeting is about and 2) reinforcing for the subject the serious nature of the meeting. Using the most objective data early has several advantages: It can set a tone, and it may reduce the chance that the impaired professional will bolt from the room or attempt to take control at the onset of the intervention.

Some examples of appropriate comments by Team Member 1 are:
1. "John, as Chief of Surgery and as your friend, I've worked with you for five years and have always had the highest respect for you, both as a person and as a surgeon. You've consistently provided excellent care to the patients. You've shown commitment to this hospital by taking extra emergency calls and filling in for other physicians. You've given generously of your time and energy not only to patients and house staff but also to the nurses to whom you give those training seminars on surgical procedures and post-operative care. We very much appreciate what you've done. But this past two months I've observed some changes in your usual performance and have received information from the operating-room nurses, the floor nurses, and several of our colleagues that concerns me greatly." He then presents specific data and says, "John, I care about you, and seeing these changes in you worries me."
2. "Mary, as your head nurse I've always admired your clinical competence and your dedication to the patients. Over the last three years you've shown great professional growth and have been a wonderful role model for new employees. But recently you seem to isolate yourself while at work, not only from me but also from your friends and co-workers. You don't even have lunch with them anymore. Several of the

staff have come to me concerned about some things that have happened recently, and I'd like to share them with you." She presents her data.

Team Member 2: This member may be a co-worker or colleague, even a direct supervisor, but someone who has closer, more frequent contact with the subject than the manager does. As a result, the information presented will appear more subjective, although in reality it's not. This team member traditionally presents firsthand observations of behavioral changes in the person and of decline in professional performance and cites specific complaints from co-workers, colleagues, and clients or patients. This player may double as the friend or colleague of the subject; this can increase the emotional impact of the presentation to the impaired professional, since it's very difficult to ignore someone who's both a friend and a colleague.

Here's an example of a statement by a colleague or co-worker:

"John, we've worked together a long time, and through the years you've been a good friend. You've seen me through some very difficult times, and I've always felt I could count on you. But something's different about you lately. You avoid talking to me, make excuses for not playing tennis with me any more. You even avoid having lunch with me in the cafeteria." (She reads from small notebook in her lap.)

"Two weeks ago, on Wednesday the sixteenth, I was making rounds at 5 p.m., and a nurse asked me to help her read an order you had written on a gall-bladder patient. When I looked at the chart I was shocked. You had written orders for a regular diet and oral medications and left no orders for pain medication." (Normally this patient would have been allowed nothing by mouth for the first day or two—only injections for pain control as needed.) "The nurse had called you on the beeper and stated that you were slurring your words and didn't recognize the name of the patient she was referring to. I corrected the orders and tried to page you, but you didn't answer. The next day when I saw you in the operating room, you made light of the situation and said the nurse had awakened you from a sound sleep. Your response worried me. It's not like you to brush off something like that. Last Tuesday at 9 a.m. while I was scrubbing, a nurse came and asked me to check on you while you were operating. I did. You were sweating and irritable, and you had difficulty holding the instruments. When I went in to see if you needed help, you yelled at me and told me to leave you alone. I smelled alcohol on your breath. John, you've been like a brother to me. I care about you, and I'm very concerned."

Team Member 3 (Optional): It may be necessary to include a third team player to present additional significant data. This person may be classified as friend but may also meet criteria as colleague or co-worker. This person generally has even more of an emotional investment with the subject and therefore may evoke more unpredictable behavior. This team member also shares with the subject information about changes in behavior or personality, tells how that has made him or her feel, and expresses sincere concern in view of these observations. This person is usually able to communicate in a very personal way because of the personal relationship.

Here's an example of comments by a colleague or friend:

"Mary, you and I have been very close for a lot of years. You've always had a special way of sharing in my life, both in and out of work, and I love you very much. But these last several months, Mary, you've pulled away from me and seem uncomfortable around me, even at work. For no reason that made sense to me, you dropped out of the art class you used to enjoy so much. You backed out on our weekly dinners, on playing bridge on Wednesday nights, and even on the trip we planned to Florida. These used to be things that you never missed, but you haven't done any of them in months. I've felt lonely, Mary, because we always shared so many things, but lately you've avoided even talking to me. When I asked you if something was wrong, you said no.

"I've also noticed several things that concern me. Last Friday, February third, when I was covering the nursing unit for lunch, your patient, Mr. Thomas in room 210, called for pain medication. When I checked his chart, I saw that you had charted giving him a shot only one hour before. When I spoke with Mr. Thomas [a 30-year-old alert and oriented patient who had a leg fracture] he said he hadn't had a shot since 6 a.m., before we both came on duty. When I checked the narcotic signout book, you had charted that Mr. Thomas was given Demerol 75 mg at 9 a.m. and also at 11:30 a.m. That scared me, Mary.

"On Monday, February sixth, I had the same patients you had taken care of earlier on Friday, and I noticed several discrepancies on their medication records. I listed three of them:

"1. Mrs. Palmer had orders for Demerol every 4 hours. You had charted that she received doses 4 times between 8 and 2, every 2 hours.

"2. Mr. White had orders for Demerol 75 mg every 3 to 4 hours, yet you signed out 4 doses of Demerol 100 mg even though we both know there's always a box of Demerol 75 mg available.

"3. Mrs. O'Malley had been taken off Demerol on February second, yet
you signed out 4 doses to her on February fourth, as well as 3 doses
of the oral medication Percodan, which was ordered.
"Mary, I care about you, and I'm very concerned about these incidents."

4. Interpretation of the Data in Terms of Professional Practice

After sharing the data, someone with known expertise about professional
leverage needs to interpret what these documented incidents mean in relation
to the subject's ability to continue in practice within the institution, state, and
potentially within the profession. At this point the **first** statement of the
"bottom line" is heard (it will be heard twice again). The member who
assumes this responsibility may be the intervention coordinator or the
institutional administrative representative. In situations involving hospital or
agency employees, the nursing executive may assume this role if the subject
is a nurse; or the chief administrator or chief of medical staff may assume the
role if the impaired professional is a staff physician. In intervening with
private practitioners, interpreting the seriousness of the documentation is
usually the role of the professional peer assistance advocate or intervenor.

In all cases, what must be clearly stated is "Because of these incidents [or
errors or discrepancies or behavioral changes] you're placing clients [or
patients] in jeopardy," or "This reported behavior is unacceptable practice in
this hospital and involves violations of the professional practice act," or "We
know after reviewing your past evaluations and recommendations that this
isn't like you. Something has changed your ability to be the doctor [or teacher
or pharmacist or whatever] you used to be, and we'd like to help." The
message here must be a double-edged sword: 1) In view of this information
we can't allow you to continue practicing, but 2) we're not only willing to
help, but we really want to help, which is demonstrated by our being here in
this room and caring enough to tell you face-to-face what we've seen and what
we want to help you do.

In cases where you have actual documentation of intoxication or of
alcohol/other drug use while on duty (such as the odor of alcohol on the breath,
slurred speech, or staggering gait) or have observed the subject taking
medication from the patient supply or narcotic cupboard, you may choose to
refer to the suspected alcohol/other drug problem when presenting the
professional interpretation to the subject. When the incidents are clearly
documented, it's safe to say, "In view of this information, we'd like you to
submit to an evaluation at one of the three chemical dependence treatment

centers we've listed here," or "Because of the observations of your colleagues, we'd like you to submit voluntarily to an evaluation at a chemical dependence treatment center, and you may choose from one of the following."

The subject clearly knows the connection between the alcohol/other drug use and the intervention, because that was the documentation presented. There are of course advantages and disadvantages in mentioning the potential chemical dependence problem, depending on the documentation available and the degree of illness of the impaired professional.

Be wary of relying too heavily on alcohol on the breath or on isolated episodes with only one witness. We found an alcoholic psychologist obviously drunk and reeling down the hall but foolishly called no one else to witness the spectacle. In spite of a solid reputation as someone unlikely to lie, this lone witness was disposed of with ease. "Yes, of course I was a bit unsteady. I know I was, and I was already on the way home. I was dead tired and trying to work in spite of a miserable cold. The antihistamine made me unsteady, and the alcohol you smelled on my breath was there all right, but it was from an alcohol-based cough syrup."

But several different witnessed incidents of intoxication are difficult to rationalize or deny, and the professional may feel forced into agreeing to the evaluation. Since acknowledging the chemical dependence is very painful, the impaired professional may well submit to the evaluation but still show righteous indignation that you could possibly think such a thing and also may become extremely defensive: "You're calling me a drunk?" or "I'm not the only one in this room who ever came to work after taking a drink" or "You think I'd stoop to stealing drugs?" This attitude can interfere with gaining closure on the intervention and may necessitate a repeat of all the documentation and the reason for requesting the evaluation. Most subjects, though, will eventually comply.

Where there's no clear documentation of actual alcohol/other drug use or diversion on duty, or no DWI charge to add significant meaning to the observed problems with professional performance, we advise that you don't address the suspected drug use. The impaired professional is already alert to any insinuation that the intervention is based on his or her alcohol/other drug use, and if you don't have adequate documentation, stating or implying such a suspicion only complicates the process. If subjects believe a case is being built against them in relation to diverting drugs or using alcohol, they usually spend their energies trying to disprove the charge. When the focus isn't fixed on the drug but on performance and behavior, the subject is considerably less defensive and more amenable to a resolution. But it still won't be easy.

If the team members decide not to address formally the suspected problem, they should prepare a rationale for why they want the person evaluated by a chemical dependence expert or at a chemical dependence treatment center. Ideally, we relay to the professional that there are certain clinicians or centers that are qualified to evaluate professionals who are showing signs of unsafe or questionable practice and that the standard procedure includes several elements: medical, psychological, psychiatric, and chemical dependence assessments. When the evaluation is complete, we explain, recommendations are then made by the evaluators for follow-up or treatment; the fact that this occurs in a chemical dependence facility really is inconsequential. This explanation usually isn't questioned except by those desperate few who try to negotiate their own evaluation with someone else, often a trusted enabler who will rescue them from this nightmare.

5. Making Recommendations and Presenting Alternatives

This role is usually assumed by the team member possessing the most authority, whether it be professional or a combination of professional and employment leverage. At this point we get to the **second** statement of the "bottom line" (it comes up one more time); we reveal exactly what we expect to have done about this situation. We've defined our leverage primarily as licensure; now we let the professional know what he or she must do to protect that licensure: "In view of the information we've shared with you here, we're recommending an immediate evaluation at a chemical dependence treatment facility," or "After reviewing all the information presented here today, we can't allow you to continue practicing until you've had a comprehensive evaluation to determine your ability to do so safely," or "In order for you to continue practicing in this agency [hospital, firm], we're requesting an evaluation at an approved treatment facility." Note that our goal is **evaluation**.

Then we state the expected time frame for following this request. "We've notified these centers, and all are prepared to admit you after this meeting," or "Arrangements have been made for you to leave for the center now, and Harry has offered to drive you home and help you pack a few things." It's crucial to reassure people at this point about their status in regard to benefits, insurance coverage, and maintenance of their position during the evaluation period. It's important, too, that individual team members restate their positive regard for the subject both as a person and as a professional.

6. Support from a Colleague in Recovery

This fellow professional is often the only advocate accepted by the impaired professional. All the others seem to be threatening the subject with incriminating data, seem to have a vested interest in building a case against him or her. And when some impaired professionals pick up the slightest hint that we're making the outrageous charge that they have a problem with alcohol/other drugs (even where there's solid documentation from narcotic records, incidents of drinking at work, observed intoxication or physical changes), they may react violently by jumping up, shouting insults, perhaps threatening team members, even throwing a chair or an ashtray.

At this point, a person in recovery may be the one who can turn the tide. Such persons may clearly identify themselves as having had the same kind of problems and as having gone successfully through the same process of intervention, evaluation, and treatment. This revelation, coupled with a friendly arm around the shoulder and some kindly words of understanding, reassurance, and promise of support, can establish real rapport and hope—the feeling that "Well, I have at least **one** friend here, someone who understands me."

7. Repetition of Concerns and Data If Necessary

In preparing your script be aware that information must often be repeated several times to the subject before it sinks in. Remember, the impaired professional is very anxious in this situation and may at first block out what you're saying. The team members should be told in advance that they may have to go around more than once .

8. "Bottom Line" Statement by Authority Figure

This is the bottom line of the bottom line. The employer, peer assistance representative, or other person who represents authority restates clearly that the person is expected to enter a designated center for evaluation. This person also presents the subject with the consequences of choosing not to follow the recommendations. The "or else" is usually the threat of licensure action through formal complaint procedures. By this point there usually isn't much of a protest if the intervention has been conducted properly. Realizing now that there really isn't any suitable alternative, subjects will almost always yield, even if they still declare their determination to clear their name or prove you wrong.

9. Closure (Contracts, Releases)

At the end of the intervention the coordinator should make a concluding statement such as "John, you've agreed to go to the treatment center today to begin the evaluation process, and you understand that until that evaluation is completed you may not practice in this facility. You also understand that you're expected to comply with the recommendations of the treatment team before you can resume your practice privileges." This clarifies for all participants exactly what the recommended procedure and agreements are. At this point the subject signs contract forms (in peer assistance programs) and/or release forms to allow the peer assistance advocate or hospital administrator to communicate with the evaluation team and later to be apprised of what is recommended. Not all programs or facilities have developed these contracts, but it's advisable to have a prepared written statement outlining the reasons for requesting evaluation and an agreement clause to be signed by the impaired professional. (See Appendix B.)

The coordinator should see to it that a release form that gives the peer assistance program or hospital permission to discuss relevant data with the treatment facility is signed at the time of intervention or as soon afterward as possible if the professional is under the influence and unable to execute a valid release. Otherwise there's always confusion about issues of confidentiality, since critical data may then not be available to the evaluating center, which in turn may not be able to communicate with the employer or peer assistance staff. Without the data about exactly what precipitated the impaired professional's need for evaluation, the treatment team may be unable to make an accurate assessment of the extent or even the nature of the problem. It certainly can't rely on the distorted perspective of the impaired professional or of an enabling family system. Understanding the subject's need for ever-stronger denial, we must provide the evaluating center with the facts.

The coordinator should also ensure compliance with required reporting mechanisms within the state. There's no need for employers ever to know the intimate details of treatment; these can and should be kept entirely confidential. They can legitimately know, however, what has been suggested about the number and type of treatment sessions. There should also be an agreement that employers can be informed if the subject doesn't honor these recommendations or fails to complete treatment. If there's mandatory reporting of impaired professionals, then the hospital, agency, or professional identifying the problem must file a report with the regulatory board. Also, if there's a state-level regulatory program requiring all chemically dependent professionals to be reported or referred to it, the subject should be encouraged to make that contact by phone before leaving the intervention.

Although some state statutes have mandatory reporting laws regarding unsafe practice, enrollment in regulatory programs is usually voluntary and must be initiated by the subject. On the other hand, peer assistance programs not operated under the licensing board may receive referrals from others besides the subject and may even attempt to locate the person and offer advocacy while getting him or her into a treatment program and including him or her in the peer assistance program itself.

In general, the coordinator should have ready access to local and state-level resources, know the statutory and professional obligations involved, and be prepared to explain these programs to the subject and to point out the advantages of participating.

As they walk through the script, team members will become less guarded emotionally and more willing to express their feelings. This is a positive effect of the small-group process. The more the team members can talk openly together, express concerns, and identify feelings, the more they'll be in touch with their individual responses to the situation and feel secure with one another. If they can unburden themselves of unfamiliar or frightening feelings, they'll be much more effective. Some will disclose very personal information during this process and will seek acceptance from the group. This is like other crisis situations we experience, whether in a community disaster, in a family, or in a hospital setting. People cooperate in meeting the immediate crisis and while doing so feel a closeness to those who are working with them. If you've ever been involved in a hospital crisis or other disaster—be it coping with multiple auto-accident victims, major fires, a subway derailment, a serious lawsuit, or even just waiting with a small group to take an important exam—you can remember how you became a kind of team and how you drew together during that time. In any crisis when we're faced with the unfamiliar, our insecurities tend to surface, and we need to help one another feel a little less vulnerable. In the small-group setting, this happens because we're not alone. We have support, reassurance, and validation of our natural fears and anxieties from others who are feeling much the same as we are—as the following brief story illustrates.

In preparing for an intervention with an attorney, a team comprised of three attorneys and a trainee intervenor met to review data and rehearse the intervention. After preparing the script and assigning roles, and while waiting for the intervention to take place, the coordinator asked the other team members nervously, "We have enough documentation, right? We really are sure about this, right?" This was the person who had initiated the intervention process! The other team members reassured him and reviewed the facts.

During this waiting period of several hours, each of the team members almost in a kind of rotation exhibited signs of anxiety. But when the subject finally did appear, the team treated him firmly but gently, and each team member was able to speak calmly and with conviction.

Establishing Ground Rules

Before the rehearsal, it's important for the team to know these guidelines to follow during the intervention.

1. Listening Without Interrupting

If the subject interrupts a team member, the coordinator will repeat the rules and explain again that the subject will have ample time to question and respond after the members have shared their concerns. For now, he or she is asked to listen.

2. Body Posturing

Members should be asked to remain in an open posture during the intervention. Crossing the legs, folding the arms, rolling the eyes, clenching the fists, or exchanging glances with other team members can all be interpreted as defensive, even hostile, gestures indicating that the team members are closed to any explanations. The subject will instinctively be searching for anything to support his or her feeling that this intervention is an attack. Also alert team members to their unconscious nervous habits: tapping a foot, biting fingernails, even chewing gum. These innocent activities can be very distracting during the intense intervention process and sometimes are seen by the impaired professional as uncaring, aggressive, or even hostile.

There should be no drinking, eating, or smoking by team members during the intervention, not only because it's distracting, but also because it suggests a casual social environment that can undermine the serious intent of the intervention.

3. Eye Contact

Eye contact is a powerful form of communicaton. When attempting to gain the full attention of the subject, as in summarizing what has been documented and spelling out its professional import, the coordinator or assigned person should keep full eye contact with the subject. This action is emphatic, even a little intimidating, but it tends to get the person focused on the seriousness of the meeting, which is exactly what's needed. If this eye contact is maintained, the subject is less likely to attempt to disrupt the intervention by inviting sympathy from a friend or other team member.

It's helpful, too, if the professional in recovery maintains direct eye contact with the subject as a way of giving gentle, nonverbal signs of acceptance and support.

On the other hand, persons who are emotionally vulnerable to the subject, either because of established personal relationships or because of possible personal intimidation, should be advised not to make direct eye contact, particularly while presenting data. The subject will frequently attempt to interrupt, trying to get the presenter to look at him or her, saying essentially, "How could you do this to me?" and may embark on numerous other attempts to get the team member to sympathize and perhaps even rescue the subject from the whole situation. Even the slightest eye contact at this point can destroy the objectivity that should accompany presentation of the data and can distract and upset the team member. It's not easy to speak to someone without looking directly at him or her, but in this case it's imperative. It's wise to have notes in hand and to look at them while speaking.

4. Seating Arrangements

Seating for the intervention is ideally in a circle, which not only affords a closed group environment but also allows team members to see each other easily for needed glances of support. It also allows for strategic placement of the subject. This circle should be large enough that members aren't jammed together and the subject doesn't feel trapped.

Never let the subject take the seat by the door; much better the seat farthest from it. If the subject becomes extremely volatile, upset, angry, or hostile, we don't want to provide an easy opportunity for the subject to slip out the door without having understood the full import of the situation and being aware of the options. Nor of course do we want the subject to leave the intervention distressed or intoxicated or to drive a car or do anything else unwise or dangerous.

Certain positions are particularly advantageous to certain team members. The person who's most vulnerable emotionally (who should avoid eye contact with the subject) should be seated immediately next to him or where it's very difficult to have direct eye contact.

Sitting nearby is a good position for the person who will hand copies of certain documents to the subject to review as data is being presented.

The person with the most leverage should sit directly across from the subject for maximum power of presence and direct eye contact.

The professional in recovery should sit right next to the subject, within arm's reach, to offer support and calming reassurance—to be literally as well as figuratively "on the same side" as the subject.

5. Safety Precautions

The intervention team also should be aware of safety precautions to be taken for the sake of all involved. The subject may be carrying weapons, so we should request that all personal belongings be left well out of reach or outside the room. (In some situations, one may even need to ask about weapons. We knew of an attorney who kept a gun in his briefcase at all times, planning to use it on himself if what he saw as an already-miserable existence got even worse.) One team member should be assigned to make emergency notifications of security personnel, psychiatric staff, or police if necessary and to have their phone numbers at hand prior to the intervention. You might also want to assign a team member to clear the room of unnecessary loose objects that can be thrown in anger or helplessness. (Heavy ashtrays have been known to fly; a subject who chain-smokes isn't likely to question why you've provided a lightweight plastic one.) Although these occurrences are rare, they can happen, so it's best to eliminate the possibility altogether.

6. Privacy and Freedom from External Interruptions

The intervention coordinator should ensure total privacy either by notifying the secretary responsible for scheduling use of the room or by posting a "Conference in Progress" sign on the door. All participants should sign out to their beeper services and paging operators and have someone else take their calls, because there should be no interrupting once the process begins. Even the slightest interruption may destroy the momentum and give the subject an opportunity to collect himself or herself and quickly build stronger defenses.

Do's and Don'ts of Intervention	
Do	*Don't*
1. Express positive regard for the subject's skills, abilities.	1. Argue.
	2. Threaten.
2. Express feelings of sincere care and concern for the person's well-being.	3. Diagnose or judge.
	4. Use judgmental tone of voice.
	5. Express anger or frustration.
3. Remain calm.	6. Demand a confession.
4. Use soft but firm, audible tone of voice.	

Rehearsing the Intervention

Now we're ready to rehearse the intervention.

We recommend that the rehearsal take place the day of the intervention itself, preferably immediately beforehand, since stress levels are often so high that a rehearsal even one day before is forgotten. Anxiety can interfere with our ability to remember even the simplest instructions, and we've found that the closer to the event the actual rehearsal is, the better the team's performance.

In setting up this rehearsal, someone must play the role of subject. Usually we ask for a volunteer. This process is interesting. Often the team member who's having the most difficulty with the anticipated intervention will volunteer to play this role and in so doing will often reveal his or her own ambivalence. For example, this person may be angry at the impaired professional for stealing from a client, stealing drugs, or forging a colleague's name but may also feel that the professional deserves an opportunity to get help by way of the intervention. Once the member has revealed this ambivalence, the group is able to discuss it and help the team member resolve it.

Speaking as if they were the subject of the intervention can often help team members get in touch with what they're really feeling about the intervention and/or about the impaired professional. Team members who have expressed resentment, verbally and otherwise, before playing the role of the subject have been quite surprised at how sympathetic they suddenly feel toward the subject. This is certainly an added benefit from the rehearsal process!

You as coordinator should outline clearly for the team exactly what will happen and when, first walking them through the outline we've presented and including the statements to be made about the purpose of the meeting. With all the team players assigned their respective roles, including the member who will play the part of the subject, you will need to:

1. Arrange the intervention seating.
2. Distribute copies of records and other documentation to be used.
3. Check each team member's script.
4. Explain again the purpose of the intervention.
5. Remind the team of what and what not to do and say during the intervention.

The rehearsal should begin just as the intervention will, with the subject arriving and the coordinator making appropriate responses and introductions. The coordinator should prompt each member when it's time to speak:

"And now, Mary, would you please share your observations and concerns with John?"

As this role play progresses it will be evident to the coordinator that some players need further coaching and that others will need extra support and reassurance throughout the intervention process. Ideally, during this rehearsal the member who plays the role of the subject will try to take on the characteristic behaviors of a person who has just been confronted with negative feedback about professional performance. These imagined responses will of course often be different during the process of intervention and can change rapidly, so the team should be prepared to respond (or not respond) appropriately. Some of the characteristic behaviors may include expressions of anger, denial, tears, pleading, hostility, attempts at manipulation, and threats toward those participating. For instance, "You can't be serious. All my evaluations have been very positive." "I can't believe you're doing this to me, Mary. I thought you were my friend." So prepare your team for all possible behaviors. You'll undoubtedly experience more than one!

The key to helping the members remain sufficiently detached from the subject's behavior (but not from the person) is simply to warn them to expect it. Remaining calm despite tears or angry outbursts will protect them from being manipulated emotionally and help them keep the intervention on course. After the rehearsal, team members should have time to talk together to discuss their perceptions, observations, and feelings about what just transpired. Again, this is an opportunity for group process to take over; members will provide support for one another.

After this group debriefing, the coordinator should address any judgmental behavior or statements or other potential problems and acknowlege the team's probable anxiety about the impending intervention. The primary task of the coordinator will be to direct, support, and reassure the team members. What they're doing is difficult and requires moral courage, but it can save both a career and a life.

Chapter Highlights

A typical intervention team may include:
1. A leader/coordinator
2. Two or more colleagues
3. A supervisor or department head (who may also serve as one of the colleagues)
4. A professional in recovery

The outline for writing the intervention script is:
1. Introductions by the coordinator
2. Statement of the purpose of the meeting by the coordinator
3. Presentation of data by 1 to 3 team members (or however many)
4. Interpretation of the data in terms of professional practice
5. Presentation of recommendations and alternatives to the subject
6. Support from a colleague in recovery
7. Repetition of concerns and data if necessary
8. "Bottom line" statement by an authority figure
9. Closure

Basic ground rules for intervention are:
1. No interruptions from the subject during the presentation of data
2. No gum chewing, eating, drinking, or smoking by team members throughout the intervention
3. No crossed arms, crossed legs, tapping feet, etc., throughout the intervention
4. Direct eye contact with the subject by the coordinator or assigned person and by the professional in recovery, but not by team members whose close personal ties with the subject make them too vulnerable emotionally
5. Each participant in the assigned seat
6. No interruptions (phone calls, beepers) once the intervention begins

To review the do's and don'ts of intervention, see page 145.

Chapter 6

Phase Two:
The Actual Intervention

Ideally, the rehearsal has taken place about two hours before the actual intervention, and the team is primed. If the rehearsal was held before the day of the intervention, though, plan to spend at least one-half to one hour with the team just before the planned intervention time. They'll need reminders of all the do's and don'ts and a walk through of the script as well as last-minute encouragement and affirmation. In either case, allow the members a few minutes to freshen up beforehand so that the subject doesn't suddenly appear and catch all of you unprepared.

Arrival of the Subject

When the subject arrives at the intervention and is greeted by the coordinator, there are several predictable responses: 1) "What is this?" or 2) "What did I do?" or 3) "You can't do this to me" or 4) I don't need to sit down; I'll just stand" or 5) "You all must be crazy" or 6) "I don't need to sit here and listen to this."

Regardless of the response, be prepared to deal with it calmly and request that the subject sit with the group for just a few minutes. If the subject feels not only threatened but angry as well, you may need to state exactly how serious the meeting is and the potential consequences of not staying and listening, such as filing a report with the licensing board or involving more powerful superiors. With some persons the approach "Of course, you can leave if you want to. No one will stop you, but we'd like to speak with you a few minutes before you do" is very effective. You haven't strong-armed anyone. The subject is still free to go, but you appear less threatening, so he or she may well decide to stay and find out what you want.

Once you have the subject in the room, gesture toward the proper seat. As we've mentioned, having the subject in the proper seat is crucial. We want to be able to communicate with maximum effectiveness, so both physical proximity and a certain amount of eye contact are essential, as Chapter 5 explained. If the team is seated already, it's easy to point to the proper empty chair and ask the subject to have a seat. When rising for introductions, team members should stay firmly in place in front of their own chairs. There will be interventions in which these details won't matter, particularly if the subject is so ill that we're only going through the motions of intervention. In those cases the details will need to be repeated when the subject has been withdrawn from alcohol/other drugs. In some other cases the subject has already seen the handwriting on the wall and may give up easily with a sigh of relief. One broadcaster said, "Thank God it's finally happened!" And one time an elderly physician welcomed two members of the Physicians' Committee of the New York State Medical Society with his wife at his side and tea carefully laid out for the visitors. The committee had received a great deal of media attention at the time, and his statement after only a few words of greeting was "We knew you were coming. But what took you so long?" But these are the unusual intervention scenarios.

When we attempt to intervene with someone in a late stage of the disease, the subject's defenses are extremely high, and attempts to slip through any loophole, both literal and figurative, will occur. If you're fully prepared, though, that poses no problem.

In preparing for an intervention with a male nurse, team members had been assigned seats, had completed a very effective role play, and had armed themselves with an impressive amount of work-related data. We didn't want to alert the subject to the intervention, so his head nurse was asked to go and get him from the unit and ask him to come with her to the office to review a medication error from the previous day. When she left the group, all were seated in the appropriate chairs. However, one of the team members asked to leave the group to make a quick phone call, and when the head nurse and the subject arrived, he promptly sat down in the wrong seat, just next to the intervention coordinator. Rather than lose the timing and rhythm of events, the coordinator let the intervention proceed.

When the presentations began, the subject was disruptive, defensive, and attempted to intimidate the head nurse, who was now in his direct line of vision. The coordinator, seeing the cost of the ineffective arrangement, signaled to another team member seated directly across from the coordinator, one who had excellent eye contact with the subject, to get up and switch seats. No words were spoken, but both stood up and casually changed seats. From that point on, the intervention proceeded smoothly. Using direct eye contact with the subject, the coordinator was able to address his behavior both verbally and nonverbally.

Individual responses differ in each intervention, depending not only on the type of documentation and the degree of leverage available, but also on differences in personalities and the degree of illness. However, among several responses that appear in almost all cases are "This can't be happening to me" and "But I'm a good doctor" (teacher, pharmacist, psychologist, nurse, pastor, judge, dentist, or whatever). These persons may see themselves primarily in terms of what they do professionally: "I'm a doctor. This doesn't happen to doctors." So when we present information that's damaging to that image, they resist it. Earlier we mentioned that often the most important, sometimes the only, remaining source of pride and satisfaction the subjects have is their profession, which in turn is represented by the license to practice or appear before the bar. Subjects know who they are in terms of their professions: "I'm a nurse" (or priest, psychologist, attorney, or whatever the profession is). As the disease progresses, this identification becomes paramount in that they may have lost most other life identifications—as husband, wife, or parent—because of their chemical dependence. When they're seated in the intervention we must help them preserve their self-esteem and identity by encouraging their colleagues to express positive regard for their professional skills and abilities. The focus of intervention is to make clear that something is interfering with their ability to practice up to their usual standard, not to prove that they're bad.

It will still be very difficult for subjects to sit through the presentation of data that explains the group's purpose in intervening, since that information tells them "They think I'm incompetent. They think I'm a failure." This perception creates their overwhelming need to defend and counterbalance what's being said with statements of personal professional competence. "I've never lost a case," "Why, I'm the best nurse on that floor," "I'm the only psychologist who does his own testing and still carries a full caseload," "I'm one of the few anesthesiologists who actually see their patients before they get to the operating room," and so on. They're not really refuting the evidence; they can't. They're merely trying desperately to salvage what they can of their self-regard.

Here are some common responses from the subject:

1. "Why are you picking on me? Plenty of other people in this place do the same thing."

2. "Is it a crime to be too busy to get someone to sign off the narcotic wastes?"
3. "Are you accusing me of stealing drugs?"
4. "Those aren't my orders. Someone else must have written them."
5. "Wait until my attorney hears about this! You'll pay for this."
6. "So I had a drink one night before coming to work. Big deal! Everyone does once in a while. You have too."
7. "This is a joke. I can go upstairs and pull charts with missing signatures from lots of other nurses."
8. "This is the thanks I get for working so many hours when you're short of help."
9. "I've been under a lot of pressure lately." (Common sources of extra stress are then named.) "I'm getting divorced," "I'm studying for boards," "I'm in school full time," "Someone poisoned my dog," "I haven't been feeling well," "My ex-wife is ill and I've got the kids," "My mother died." (The list goes on and on and on but asks you to assume that chemical dependence is caused by stress and cured by its removal. Excuses of this type are usually followed by some version of "I'll do better from now on.")
10. "You can't force me to do anything. I'm innocent, and I can prove it."
11. "I can get a job anywhere."

There are or course many more lines, but they fall into these basic categories:

1. **Defiance:** "You can't do this to me," "I dare you to try and get away with this."
2. **Threats:** "You'll pay for what you've done. My attorney will hear about this," "I'll have your job for this."
3. **Denial:** "It wasn't me," "I didn't write that," "I didn't take care of that patient," "I wasn't drinking," "I didn't say that," "I have no idea what you're talking about."
4. **Excuses:** "I worked a double shift that day," "I've been sick for a couple of weeks," "I had a cold and was taking antihistamine, so that one drink I had really hit me," "I was tired after operating all night," "I was floated to that department and didn't know the patients," "My partner's been on vacation, and I guess I'm overworked," "The court was crazy that day."
5. **Promises:** "I'm really sorry that happened, but it won't happen again," "I'll be more careful next time," "I'll never do that again."
6. **Bargaining:** "I'll never drink anything before coming to work ever again, if you'll just forget this happened," "I'll go see someone I know

152

who does counseling. I know I don't need to go to that center. I'll be fine if you'll just let me work things out my way," "I'll take some leave; I guess I've been working too hard," "Just give me one more chance. You never said anything about this before. My kids are in college. I need this job."

The impaired professional may switch around among these responses or use all of them in one intervention. We must keep in mind what a threat we present as we challenge the one thing the subject thought was most stable in an otherwise out-of-control life, his or her profession. On one level, a subject knows perfectly well that what he or she is doing (using alcohol/other drugs or stealing drugs at work) is wrong, ethically and professionally, but it's a complicated matter, since the subject now needs the drug and can't stop using. On the other hand, the person can barely manage the losses the alcohol/other drug use is causing: family, friends, physical health. Now livelihood and professional identity are in jeopardy as well. So, although chemically dependent people know they're diverting drugs or practicing while intoxicated and that this is a major violation of the code of ethics of their profession, they must suppress the awareness because it's much too painful. Continuing in denial protects them from fully realizing and facing the problem.

Intervention as a Crisis

Since intervention presents a true crisis both personally and professionally, many chemically dependent professionals can't handle what they're hearing and may appear totally immobilized as they attempt desperately to ward off the blows. They hear a particularly embarrassing story or a shocking example of risk to a client and start frantically preparing a rebuttal. As their minds are busy with this, they hear only parts or perhaps none of the other data. What they hear us saying is "If you don't face and deal with what appears to be an alcohol/other drug problem, we'll turn you over to the authorities." So as they see it, we've placed them in a position where there's really no choice that doesn't appear agonizing at best. They're not willing to give up their livelihood or the profession they've worked so hard to serve, but they may panic at the thought of having to stop using alcohol/other drugs. This developing anguish in the subject is frequently observed in the intervention process as progressive disorganization.

Progressive Disorganization

Subjects react with a host of defenses: They can't hear what's being said; they interrupt, rationalize, lash out at those around them, projecting blame onto everyone and everything but themselves. They may lose control and have violent outbursts of temper. Regardless of how they react, it's critical that you not get upset and that you set limits in a calm, reassuring way. They should be allowed to express their feelings, but not in a potentially harmful way. They must be redirected to take their seats, offered quiet but firm direction, and have limitations set on their behavior. It's very helpful at this point to offer support and empathy by calmly listening for a brief period without argument; this often subdues the subject's feeling of powerlessness. The crisis we've precipitated must remain purposeful and lead to resolution. The subject undoubtedly feels both helpless and hopeless and needs support and direction from both coordinator and group.

There will be instances when disorganization isn't evident as the subject maintains a rigid, stoic posture, but it's there. When the subject constantly questions the team and focuses on things other than the data presented or ignores major parts of it, you'll realize he or she hasn't heard what's been said. The team members must simply repeat the data collected and their individual concerns for him or her. Be patient. This should be done matter-of-factly, not in an "I-already-told-you-and-why-weren't-you-listening?" way. After all, if something hasn't been heard, it's perfectly reasonable to present it again. Usually this second round is successful, at least in getting the subject to understand the objective nature of the intervention data. Even if not everything registers, the subject will probably hear enough to get the point.

Grieving

Intervention tells impaired professionals that they risk losing several things of great value to them. First, they may perceive an impending loss of professional reputation, stature, or perhaps even privileges, all of which pose a great threat of losing the image they've had of themselves. Secondly, they may connect some of the data presented to their use of alcohol/other drugs and sense that those drugs too will be taken away. Thirdly, people who are important to the impaired professional are participating in what subjects see as a damaging attack upon them personally. In their distorted perceptions, they feel the immediate loss of once-valued friendships. In this situation, most people really can't work through or even totally comprehend the impact of all these losses, and they tend to respond in stages that resemble the grief process described by Elisabeth Kübler-Ross: denial, anger, bargaining, depression, and finally acceptance. The process she describes often takes weeks or months to complete when dealing with death, but we've all experienced losses on a much smaller scale that we resolve in hours or days, depending on their magnitude. If we've lost a favorite piece of jewelry or tennis racket, we go through a much-shortened version of this same grieving process, ultimately reaching acceptance that we no longer have the ring or the tennis racket—and we move on. Losses do occur, even on a daily basis, and we work through those same processes over and over to regain equilibrium.

As we've noted, impaired professionals at the time of intervention may already have suffered significant losses and are now facing more. So they often respond by going through the following stages of grieving:

Stage One: Denial. Denial, or refusing to accept painful reality, is already present as part of the chemical dependence, but now it's fortified with denial based on additional perceived losses. Subjects attempt to explain each event or incident to convince the team and themselves that the whole thing is a mistake. They may even flatly refuse to acknowledge their own handwriting on charts, memos, or narcotic records. They aren't simply lying. They may sincerely believe what they're saying, no matter how implausible it is. They're attempting to deny the loss of professional competence. This denial becomes even more evident when specific information about the alcohol/ other drug use is presented. Then they may attempt to rationalize, blame, minimize, justify, or intellectualize even more in an effort to maintain their own unstated belief that their drug of choice is a solution, not a problem, and that they need it to keep on functioning.

Stage Two: Anger. When constantly faced with objective data about their behavior and performance, subjects may move into overt anger. How dare you threaten the things that are the most important to them! This anger is expressed to individual team members more often than to the group as a whole and perhaps focuses on those who seem the most vulnerable, their friends. When friends are perceived as traitors, it's natural for impaired professionals to ventilate their anger toward them: "Mary, how can you do this to me? I thought you were my friend!" After what they perceive as betrayal, anger is almost a necessary part of the grieving process. When people die it isn't unusual for us to become angry, even at them. After all, their death has caused us tremendous pain, and we can't at that point differentiate between the cause of the actual loss and the fact that the person has abandoned us. Similarly, these impaired professionals are struggling to maintain balance while, it seems, we're bent on stripping them of all their supports.

This self-protective anger is the basis for some of the defiance, projection, and threats we may see. Understanding that it's a normal part of coming to grips with reality places the behavior in a framework of expected and reasonable reactions. We mustn't take it personally and above all mustn't react with anger and counterattacks of our own. We're the ones in the position of strength. We can afford to be kind, and we certainly don't need to get defensive because of any unworthy motives attributed to us or accusations of unfairness. We must ignore the name-calling and stay focused on the goal.

Stage Three: Bargaining. Impaired professionals make many attempts at bargaining during the intervention and the subsequent treatment process. Realizing the full impact of what's at stake, they strive to reduce the distress and minimize the losses by attempting to manipulate the situation. During intervention we often see partial compliance and an admission that there might be a little problem, but subjects try to decide for themselves what action is appropriate—something that seems to them less painful and certainly something less definitive than what you have in mind. They may try to determine the place and circumstances of the evaluation, which certainly won't be one of the treatment centers you recommend. Subjects often seek delay and therefore propose a contract with the team to watch their behavior for a month to see if there are any more problems; if there are, **then** they may try asking you to forget some of the incriminating data to reduce the likelihood of disciplinary action, in return for which they'll go to treatment. But they're merely trying to salvage some personal control over the situation and to create a situation less potentially damaging to themselves.

They'll usually make every effort to persuade you that it will be enough for them to do much less than what you indicate they should do—something that leaves them still at work, with minimal disruption of schedules while they go through the motions of seeing someone on an outpatient basis.

A nurse was discovered to have a longstanding Demerol addiction. She was injecting at least thirty cc's a day and supplementing that with sedatives and tranquilizers. The board agreed with her that she could be seen twice a week in individual treatment at a mental health clinic that had little or no expertise in treating chemical dependence. When this ill-advised plan failed, it was blamed on the nurse, who was labeled "not motivated," and her license was revoked. She's still lost to the nursing profession.

Stage Four: Depression. If the impaired professional has already sustained major losses (e.g., a divorce, problems with the children, poor physical health) prior to intervention, he or she may already be grieving and showing signs of depression. If a person is depressed at the time of intervention and shows none of the other stages of grief, this may indicate a much more serious problem. Depression is common in the late stages of chemical dependence, but nevertheless a person will usually exhibit the common defenses when confronted. Those who sit quietly at an intervention and don't respond to anything said are clearly at high risk. Such people quite understandably feel helpless—powerless to change what has happened or to retrieve what they've lost. Now they must also face the work of recovery, a major change that takes great energy—and they have little of it left. Professionals in this stage of hopelessness will usually go along unquestioningly with any recommendation made. In chemical dependents, feeling depressed is very common, although they may at first exhibit the depression in different ways. When they're first admitted to treatment, it's very hard to distinguish between current grief, delayed grief, sadness, despair, reactive depression, other affective disorders, and the direct physiological effects of alcohol/other drug use. Usually after safe withdrawal from alcohol/other drugs, some of the depression begins to disappear, but it's wise initially to treat these persons as clinically depressed until things can be sorted out by a skilled professional, something that may be impossible to do until the period of withdrawal has passed.

Stage Five: Acceptance. Many intervention teams do get to see acceptance by the impaired professional, not necessarily the acceptance of a diagnosis of chemical dependence, but acknowledgment of the situation and how serious it is. These professionals admit and assume responsibility for the problem and accept the need for evaluation and treatment. Despite their denial that the dependence really happened, their anger that it happened, their bargaining, and their sadness and longing for what's gone, they're powerless to turn back the clock. They do realize that their situation is nonnegotiable if the intervention team doesn't waver, and eventually many do accept that fact.

On the other hand, compliance (outward acceptance with hidden reservations) can really be attributed more to the anger stage but achieves the goal of intervention anyway. The difference is that professionals who can begin working through the grieving process during intervention arrive at the treatment center in a considerably more stable emotional state. Of course, they still face the true grieving process of giving up alcohol/other drugs permanently, but they manage some resolution of the crises surrounding the intervention. Those who leave intervention in Stage 2 (anger), still protesting and struggling, are certainly challenging to deal with, but eventually they usually follow the action plan willingly enough. In short, dealing with an angry subject is less difficult than attempting to reach a depressed one.

As the professional moves through treatment, recovery, and reintegration, the grieving process is experienced repeatedly. What we see during the intervention is an abbreviated version of what will later follow on a different scale, but we can accept the subject's need to be heard and can offer reassurance. What's really lost and what's gained in recovery usually comes as a surprise. Old friends with whom the subject had little in common other than drinking or smoking pot now seem to be rather boring and are rather spontaneously replaced by more interesting new friends. Many personal problems and physical complaints may vanish almost by magic, and long-standing depression may disappear. On the other hand, some problems that have been pushed aside by a few drinks or a few pills are now waiting and must be reckoned with. Some colleagues may reject the subject and may stop referring clients to him or her, but others will unexpectedly come forth with support and comfort. Some may unexpectedly turn out to be in recovery themselves; others will say they had been aware of the subject's problem for a long time, had been worried, and are delighted their friend is well again. Exactly how personal gains and losses will balance out is unpredictable, but the changes that inevitably occur usually bring about positive personal growth.

The Coming-to-Terms Phase

After the team members have spelled out why they're so concerned about the subject's deteriorating practice and hence why they feel intervention is necessary, the subject begins to understand that the group is truly united and firm, then typically begins to bargain and make promises. When those maneuvers fail, there's usually an apparent giving in. Remember, we've offered only two alternatives: either evaluation and treatment or being fired and being reported for potentially severe disciplinary action by the board.

A physician who for many years intervened with Catholic priests, nuns, and brothers had strong backing from the church's hierarchy. "The red hat was always floating in the air close behind me," he used to say. At the end of a discussion with a priest he'd say, "Father, thou art a priest forever, but if you refuse treatment, tomorrow you'll be an inactive priest."

This process of giving in and giving up takes place on many levels, and certainly very few impaired professionals will admit that there's a primary problem with drinking or admit to taking all those drugs. You may see compliance, but the surrender is only apparent: "I'll go just to protect my license," or on a somewhat more conciliatory level, "I guess I might need just a little help right now. Maybe I could get some counseling," or "I guess I've been drinking a little more than usual, because I'm under so much pressure."

Regardless of what level of compliance is displayed, we must accept people where they are and not push for any unnecessary confessions or disclosures. It really doesn't matter whether they use alcohol or other drugs or, in the case of other drugs, where they got them. We're concerned only with getting them into the safety of the treatment center and into the care of those who have expertise in this field. We may not be able to diagnose the chemical dependence, but we have the duty to provide the diagnosticians with as much objective information as possible. If we directly accuse the subject of diverting drugs, we'll probably get a very defensive response. So at all costs stay away from unnecessary labeling, confronting, and demanding to know. Remember that most professionals maintain a mental image of drug addicts as unemployed street people who steal to get money for drugs and are never cured. The mental picture of the alcoholic isn't much more pleasant, so this is the last thing they could be.

One pharmacist who daily swallowed near-lethal doses of narcotics in tablet form said that one reason he never injected himself was that he "didn't want to risk becoming an addict"; he was merely taking a few tablets for back pain. When we intimate that some of our observations and some of the subject's problems are related to administering drugs, signing out drugs, or having the smell of alcohol on the breath, the impaired professional will undoubtedly feel that we're judging and labeling without proof. If we don't have actual proof of the alcohol/other drug use, it's often best—as we've emphasized before—to stick to what we can prove, without insisting on agreement about the root of the problem. Another obvious reason for avoiding making the diagnosis ourselves is the possibility of litigation. Many of us don't have the expertise to diagnose chemical dependence, so even if we have sound reason to believe that it's the source of the professional's problems, or even if it seems quite obvious to us, we don't formally state that conclusion during the intervention unless we have actual proof on hand.

In a well-planned intervention with a nurse, the Director of Nursing served on the intervention team. After full preparation and role play it was evident the Director was having great difficulty accepting that the nurse could have diverted so much morphine. The narcotic records and corresponding patient charts strongly indicated diversion. All the behavioral symptoms were those usually seen in chemical dependence. There was significant documentation of medication errors, omissions in patient care, and lapses in memory. But the Director repeatedly expressed disbelief, saying, "She's an excellent nurse. I even promoted her to charge nurse last year. She can't be doing this." Unfortunately, because of the nature of the documentation and the organizational structure of the institution, the Director of Nursing was a critical team member, so we attempted to limit the focus of the intervention strictly to presenting the objective information, which indicated that this nurse wasn't meeting the usual standards of practice; hence the requested evaluation. Before the intervention, the Director appeared less preoccupied with the possible diversion, although she continued to appear anxious.

During the intervention, the presentation of data by the team was very effective, and the subject made only minimal attempts to project or to excuse her behavior. So we believed we'd have a rather short but successful intervention. Wrong! Just at the point where the nurse was beginning to capitulate, the Director said, "I need to know if you took that morphine and how much of it." She certainly didn't do this in an accusatory way; she was simply compelled by her own need to know the truth. The nurse's response was predictable. She quickly went on the defensive, indignant that anyone would even imply such a thing. Several long minutes of dialogue transpired between the Director and the nurse before we were able to interrupt their discussion and regain the nurse's attention.

We attempted to undo the damage by moving quickly away from the highly threatening label of "addict" and restating to the nurse the reason for the intervention. The coordinator calmly said, "I'm not concerned with the narcotic records. Let's just put them aside. I'm concerned with these medication errors [describing each one], these omissions in patient care [discussing each one], and these reports of your outbursts in the patient-care area, your arguing with physicians, and the like. These incidents tell me that something is interfering with your ability to practice. I know by the evaluations and references I've read that you're an excellent nurse with the highest standards, and yet these recent events tell me something has changed. That's why we're requesting the evaluation: to learn what the problem is, get you some help, and bring you back to work when it's been resolved." The nurse responded well to the less threatening presentation of information and soon agreed to the evaluation.

While she was in treatment we found out that she had diverted the morphine and had reached the point in her disease where her physical tolerance was extremely high. Her obvious need for medication to prevent serious withdrawal symptoms early in her treatment, plus the multiple injection sites discovered through a physical exam, verified the diagnosis. But if we had insisted on confirming our suspicions during the intervention, she might well have rejected our recommendations altogether.

During the coming-to-terms phase of the intervention, we must clearly outline our expectations for the impaired professional:
1. What exactly do we want the person to do?
2. Where will this be done, and for how long?
3. Under what conditions may there be a return to work? What must be done to maintain benefits?
4. If there's mandatory reporting, when and to whom must it be done?
5. If there's to be enrollment in a peer assistance or regulatory program, when and how will this take place?

The most effective means of reinforcing our expectations is through a prepared program treatment contract that includes all the preceding information plus any necessary releases. There is then a permanent record of what has just taken place. In retrospect people may be or pretend to be confused about what was agreed on or about what really happened, so this contract documents exactly what the agreements are on both sides. This contract can be a most effective tool if the subject later attempts to manipulate the treatment system or disputes the need for continuing treatment. The contract should clearly state that all the recommendations of the professional treatment team regarding treatment and therapies are to be followed to the letter. This contract may be used to advantage if a second intervention is needed. (Samples of contracts of this type are included in Appendix B.)

Ideally, the impaired professional is given a choice among at least three sites for the evaluation. In the preparation phase you identified centers approved by your state-level programs. If you have a wider choice, choose centers with demonstrated, not just claimed, expertise in treating chemically dependent people. A center's experience in treating members of this particular profession is desirable, but a special program for each occupational group has never been proven to be better than having a greater mix in treatment. Some, in fact, feel that a major problem of some professional groups such as healthcare professionals is their habit of clannishness, so that they have increasing difficulty interacting with others. If this is true, it would be unwise to reinforce that tendency in treatment.

As we've already discussed, you should include one center geographically removed from your own community or state. (Remember that in these days of air travel, distance can be measured in hours, not in miles.) Affording impaired professionals the chance to decide which center to use is reassuring, since many subjects conclude that everyone feels them to be incompetent. Once the place is chosen, they should be helped to develop a task-oriented action plan that will help them organize the next few hours and smooth the transition into evaluation and treatment.

The action plan should be simple but should leave the impaired professional free to make some choices and have some feeling of control in the situation. It might include:

1. Choosing one of the three acceptable centers (a choice made before leaving the intervention)
2. Notifying family, close friends, significant others
3. Securing a colleague to cover professional obligations
4. Taking a quick look at the appointment calendar for social obligations, appointments with tradespeople, dental appointments that may need to be canceled or postponed
5. Making arrangements for child care, pets, property management, bill paying, etc.
6. Packing some personal belongings for the stay at the center

The impaired professional can use this opportunity to regain some sense of competence both in decision making and in mastering the task at hand. Not only does this improve morale, but the subject begins to make some personal investment in carrying out the recovery project. The subject who is entirely passive and resentful while others arrange everything is more prone to look for ways to sabotage the project or to escape. You can help the impaired professional make this plan immediately after he or she agrees to the recommendations, while the group is still present. Group members, particularly if they're friends of the subject, will be able to offer help in completing some of the tasks outlined above, or they may merely offer to stay with the impaired professional and escort him or her to the treatment facility.

This is the time when all the good motives that impelled associates of the professional to engage in destructive enabling behavior can be turned into assets. The caretakers can set about taking care of the cat, making explanations to clients, patients, or parishioners, even helping in the law office. In the past, such actions were counterproductive, since they served only to teach the impaired person that someone else would take care of his or her responsibilities. Now these kindly actions can really smooth the road to recovery and help the subject regain health instead of encouraging denial, cover-up, and avoidance of treatment.

The Risk of Suicide

After the subject has signed the contract and agreed to the action plan, and after you've notified the treatment center and the peer assistance or other program, the subject should if possible not be left alone. This is a critical period where the risk of suicide is very real. We recommend not intervening with anyone until all needed systems are ready to roll. A bed should be available at each of the three potential treatment centers, and some designated support person should be on hand to stay with and help the subject with tasks to be done immediately after the intervention and then with transportation to the treatment center.

Remember that people we've intervened with probably were already in trouble, and we've now compounded that trouble. The secret is out, or soon will be. The subject may feel exposed, ashamed, overwhelmed.

Subjects probably won't have these feelings very long, since with good treatment will come a whole new understanding about chemical dependence and what it really means. They'll find there's every reason for optimism, that recovery is not only possible but probable, and that part of recovery will be a renewed sense of self-worth and enjoyment of life. Even though we know these things, the person just coming out of an intervention can no more believe them than someone just abandoned unexpectedly in the midst of a love affair can believe that the pain will pass and he or she will find a new love. It doesn't seem that life will ever again be worth living. In such a situation, suicide doesn't seem unreasonable to the subject. Most of the women who were intervened with have said that they did contemplate suicide, not once but several times during their time of active chemical dependence, and some did so afterward as well. One dangerous period was immediately after intervention, another in the first few days of treatment when the sense of defeat was overwhelming and before the pain had been replaced by a realistic optimism and confidence in the future. Many say that even while accompanied by someone supportive, they tried to get rid of that person just for a few minutes in order to get to a stash of drugs or a gun, or to get into the car alone and drive off the bridge.

While lecturing at a workshop in another state we asked the peer assistance coordinator for the state-level program to do a presentation on her program to a nursing management group and to help with intervention training the next day. During the first day of the workshop, she told us about an intervention at a local hospital that involved a nurse suspected of diverting drugs.

Frequent discrepancies in the narcotic records, as well as other complaints, had been brought to the attention of the head nurse, who with the director decided that the peer assistance coordinator should be consulted. The peer assistance coordinator was shown the records and, not surprisingly, discovered discrepancies in the narcotic records not only for Demerol but also for morphine, Valium, Talwin, and several other drugs. In all, there were 156 documented discrepancies between the narcotic signout records, patient charts, and doctors' orders. Several friends who worked with the suspected nurse told of her borrowing medications from other units and of her unpredictable moods. One described how the nurse on one occasion was so disoriented that she couldn't even find her way out of the hospital. Yet no one reported the incident. The complete data showed the classic symptoms of chemical dependence.

An intervention was carefully planned, rehearsed, and carried out, but the nurse remained indignant, denied that anything was amiss, and flatly refused to cooperate with an evaluation. At the time of intervention she appeared lucid and coherent but resisted all attempts to persuade her to enter an evaluation center.

After the intervention, the coordinator requested that the nurse call her boyfriend to tell him what had happened and what the team was requesting of her, hoping he would confirm her need for treatment. She did tell him what they wanted her to do but merely said they'd discuss it when she got home. Sensing a stalemate, the coordinator repeated to the nurse that she must submit to the evaluation to avoid disciplinary action by the nursing board, urged her to discuss this with her boyfriend, and asked that she call in her decision sometime the next day. She was given phone numbers of many persons to contact in the interim, including 24-hour beeper numbers of people available to her, and the intervention concluded at 2 p.m.

The next morning the nurse came to the hospital and asked to speak with the Director of Nursing. She sat down in the Director's office, pulled a gun from her purse, and shot herself in the head.

We can never prevent all suicides of chemically dependent people, but we can take two important steps in that direction. One is to **stress early intervention by colleagues**. It's sad to think of how many good professionals take their own lives long before colleagues even attempt intervention. We need to emphasize that chemically dependent people are victims of a disease that can only grow worse if untreated. The situation is especially ironic for impaired healthcare professionals allowed to die while surrounded by the very people who should be best able to diagnose their problem and get them into treatment.

We do stress intervention **by colleagues**. Reporting the subject to authorities and leaving it to them is of course much easier on us. But state agencies simply aren't equipped to spend much time, money, and effort preventing suicides. That leaves it up to us.

The second major step we can take to prevent suicides, then, is to **be alert to certain danger signals and take certain precautions** as we prepare an intervention.

1. Is there any verbal expression of suicidal intent now? Was there in the past?

2. Is the subject suddenly very complacent, even cheerful, about the impending admission for evaluation?

3. Does the subject plan to drive home alone after the intervention? (Even if there's no obvious sign of upset, avoid this.)

4. When there's to be a stop at home, stay with the subject at all times. (More things than clean clothes are kept in dresser drawers, and we don't know what may be in the medicine cabinet.)

5. Don't permit unescorted trips to the office or unit. Have someone else get whatever was left behind.

6. If you suspect there's a supply of alcohol/other drugs at home, encourage admission to the treatment center directly from the intervention site and let someone else collect the subject's personal belongings. While the subject is in treatment, tell the family how to look for alcohol/other drugs hidden in the home. (Uncovering them, like hiding them, is a real art. Ask any person in recovery.)

7. If the center chosen requires a plane trip, there are several ways to ensure safety. Some state-level regulatory programs will book the flight reservations and secure seats for two persons: the subject and an escort. This is common practice in some programs and can be coordinated with the treatment center, which sends someone to the airport to meet and escort the subject to the center. In other cases, subjects make their reservations, usually at their own expense, and are encouraged to have a family member or friend go with them to the center. When this isn't possible because of money problems or because no other escort is available, a team member or professional in recovery can accompany the subject to the airport, put him or her on the plane, and see to it that someone from the treatment center meets the subject on arrival. Don't leave the boarding area until you're certain the plane is leaving and the subject is really aboard.

One time we carefully escorted an impaired friend onto the jetway but left the airport before the airplane door was closed. Unfortunately, the friend also left the airport. Another time, confident that now we knew all the tricks, we put a person on a plane and watched it take off but failed to notice that the flight wasn't a nonstop. We've been told of a dentist who took four days, with many stopovers, to fly from California to Minneapolis. We know from experience that most airports have several bars. In planning for chemical dependents, information of any kind is rarely wasted.

Exactly how you handle these precautions will depend on the physical and emotional condition of the subject, the individual situation, the resources available, and the recommendations of the treatment center. However, from a treatment perspective, it's quite advantageous to have a family member accompany the subject to treatment so that the treatment team can meet and hear out the family or significant others. Their participation is a critical part of any treatment program, and it should begin on the day of admission. In spite of our previous warnings, when you **can** get the cooperation of the family without sabotaging the intervention itself, do so.

We've heard wives and sweethearts of chemical dependents say, "Everyone was busy taking care of him, but no one paid any attention to me." It takes little imagination to appreciate the major upset it causes a family when a chemically dependent family member is unexpectedly whisked off to treatment. Family members may know little or nothing about chemical dependence and are now alone, upset, and frightened. Enlist the help of treatment-center staff, peer assistance people, and other professionals in recovery to ensure that the family isn't abruptly left sitting there. You've been through the whole process of learning about chemical dependence and what to do. The family has been left out of that crash course but needs that information desperately.

Wrapping up the Process

Even though your subject is being escorted to evaluation, you still have work to do:

1. Complete the documentation.
2. Complete the notifications (peer assistance, and both the treatment center chosen and those holding a bed in reserve but not finally chosen).
3. Copy the records, as appropriate, and secure them.
4. Make sure there's agreement on what co-workers are to be told about where their colleague has gone and for how long. (This point is developed in the next chapter.)
5. Provide closure for the intervention team. (This is the subject of the next chapter.)

Items 1, 2, and 3 call for brief comment.

1. In completing the documentation, you or the administrative team member may write a brief summary of the intervention, outlining the data presented about changes in the professional's practice and about

other significant behaviors. This summary statement will serve to record events objectively for future reference (for instance, to help in further treatment recommendations or to evaluate treatment options after a relapse). Memory can't be trusted for long. Also, if you have other pertinent information that wasn't used in the intervention, get this whenever possible in writing, with particular attention to date, times, and **objective** description of events. Opinions and generalities such as "He's just been looking funny for months" are of little use. If detailed objective information isn't available, at least include a carefully worded note of what has allegedly occurred so that, if need be, this data can be pursued later.

2. If notifying the regulatory agency, peer assistance, or regulatory program is required but wasn't feasible at the time of intervention, do it now while details are still easily remembered. In states where reporting is mandatory, this doesn't violate confidentiality. Relate the events as objectively as possible, and forward any requested documentation.

3. Once the records of the intervention are complete, secure them in a locked file. Where they're to be kept will depend on the nature of the intervention, the setting, and the persons involved. They're usually kept in the place of employment if the subject is employed in a healthcare facility, social-service agency, large church, law firm, or the like. If the subject is in private practice, records may be maintained by a peer assistance or regulatory program director or member of a committee for the impaired. After securing a release from the subject, the content of these records may be shared with the staff at the treatment center where the client has gone during the initial evaluation process. Never turn over the original records to the treatment center. Their staff is probably just as human as your own and just as likely to misplace things. Make sure your data is kept available (should you need it again) and safe from the idle curiosity of personnel clerks and co-workers.

Chapter Highlights

In this chapter we discussed the actual intervention process: typical responses of impaired professionals to intervention, methods of presenting the data to impaired professionals, the grief reaction of the professional, and how to help the subject by way of a short-term plan for completing tasks. Several key points of this chapter are:

Some predictable responses from impaired professionals are:
1. Defiance
2. Threats
3. Denial
4. Excuses
5. Promises
6. Bargaining

The grieving process: The impaired professional may already have suffered significant losses (such as family, friends, and physical health) before the intervention. During the intervention the subject is facing new losses and often responds by exhibiting various stages of the grieving process:
1. Denial
2. Anger
3. Bargaining
4. Depression
5. Acceptance (Initial acceptance or compliance comes when the subject agrees to the evaluation request.)

The closing statements to impaired professionals should include:
1. Exactly what we expect them to do
2. Where this will be done
3. Under what conditions they may return to work
4. If and how they will be reported to the licensing agency
5. If they must enroll in a peer assistance program
6. What the consequences will be if they don't comply with all the above
7. A request to sign needed releases

The short-term action plan for professionals after intervention should include:
1. Having them decide which of the three treatment centers they would prefer
2. Notifying family and close friends
3. Making arrangements for child care, pets, property management, paying bills, etc.
4. Packing some of the subject's personal belongings for the stay at the center

For precautions to take against the subject's possible suicide, see the list on page 165.

Chapter 7

Phase Three: Closure

The leader can now focus attention on the team members. Having completed Phase Two of intervention, team members can now relax a bit. They'll be ready to process what has happened and move toward closure. Each will have a different perspective on what took place. Each should be given the chance to express feelings, concerns, and impressions of what has occurred and to get feedback from the other group members and the leader. For many, this session will serve as a general catharsis, a process of decompression, a letting go; for others, a basic clarification of what really happened. During this session, the group process will take over and team members will usually quite spontaneously help one another sort out their perceptions and feelings.

Needs of the Team

After most interventions there are predictable responses from team members:
1. **Guilt**: "I really feel bad doing this. With three kids to support he really needs the job."
2. **Anger**: "How could she do this to us [our profession or organization or institution]?" "No really decent person could do that." "How could he just sit there and deny he did those things?"
3. **Rejection**: "I really don't care if he does get reported. It's his own fault." "He brought it on himself by messing with drugs in the first place." "He's a pharmacist. He knows better." "I really wasn't that close to her in the first place."

4. **Ambivalence**: "What if we've made a mistake?"
5. **Pessimism**: "It really looks pretty bad. He seemed like such a good therapist." "She's been in trouble for so long, and they say the prognosis isn't good for people like that." "He didn't seem to agree with what we were saying; and if he doesn't see it, how can he change?"
6. **Denial**: "I think the divorce really took its toll. Lots of people get drunk sometimes. He just needs time to get things together, maybe some counseling." "I'm sure it's not as bad as it sounds. Aren't we making a big deal of a few tranquilizers?"
7. **Hope**: "I'm glad we did this so she'll get the help she needs." "Maybe he'll be able to come back to work soon after treatment."

Although team members begin to identify and work through some of their initial feelings regarding the intervention, some may still find it difficult to resolve them, particularly those who were close to the subject and perhaps involved as enablers. These people are often guilt-ridden and very uncomfortable.

Depending on the degree of emotional involvement the team members have with the person, there may be real upset. Will the person be unforgiving? Will the friendship be lost? Was this the person from whom they've expected love, support, and understanding? Responses of team members may make for sadness and anxiety, anxiety that often surfaces in a reevaluation of the relationship they thought they had. The data presented in intervention doesn't reflect the person they thought they knew, so they may now question their ability to see other things as they really are. If their friend is impaired, how healthy is that relationship and their other relationships? Are other people dishonest and deceitful with them, while all along hiding their alcohol/other drug use? What else do they miss? While evaluating these thoughts, close friends of the colleague may now question their own failings in identifying the problem, even question their own wellness. If it could happen to someone like this, why not to them? This realization can create an overall anxiety, particularly if they've shared drinks or other drugs with their friend or colleague.

Feelings of loss are common. Long after the intervention they're still worrying about "what I should have done" and "what I shouldn't have done." Team members' reactions aren't very different from the impaired professional's own response to the intervention: a sense of personal loss. The documentation they've seen or provided has revealed the very real imperfections of a friend, perhaps a very close friend, and they begin to feel the loss of that relationship, or at least of a great part of it. After intervention you may even hear team members refer to the impaired professional in the past tense! Subconsciously they're referring to the person they used to know, not the subject they just sent off to treatment or the different one who may return. In the hearts and minds of those who deeply cared about this person there's a different image of the person they knew, someone who's now even physically removed from their world. Resolving all these feelings is a very difficult, complex matter, but the important thing to remember is that some team members will be grieving the loss of a dear friend, a loss they've helped to cause.

They may express a variety of feelings during the resolution phase, and should be encouraged to do so. The sooner they can recognize, acknowledge, and express them, the sooner they'll resolve them. Team members who have had a significant relationship with the impaired professional may need to be referred to local professionals with expertise in chemical dependence, frequently under the guise of learning a bit more about how to be most helpful to the subject during recovery. Very often it takes only one session for team members to receive a kind of absolution for their earlier denial or mismanagement; they can finally accept that they've done the best they could in the situation.

Those participants who continue to have difficulty need reassurance and will often seek it from you, the intervention coordinator, if you remain available. They may call several times to ruminate about the experience and work over the same information. Often they're helped considerably if you simply reiterate how difficult it is to identify chemical dependence, especially when one is close to the person and is trying to help. Once team members hear this message clearly, it gives them the acceptance and reassurance they need and, more importantly, the conviction that they did the right thing and can now move on.

Here's a word of caution. Don't take on a counseling role with team members. If they have significant unresolved issues, refer them to others for counseling.

Persons who hold management positions in the facility where the chemically dependent person is employed and identified will frequently have difficulty reconciling their feelings of failure in not having identified the problem sooner. As they participate in the data-collection process, what appeared at first to be a piece of isolated information often completes the puzzle and places before them a devastating total picture. After reviewing the data in its entirety, they often feel they've been stupid and have performed poorly—the situation should have been obvious long ago. Since the picture now appears so clear with all the data in hand and with the wisdom of hindsight, they blame themselves for having missed certain key indicators as soon as they occurred, perhaps weeks, months, even years ago. If this could happen, what else are they missing?

Without reassurance and support from the coordinator or someone else they trust, these management persons may judge themselves rather harshly and feel ashamed and guilty. The danger for them personally is that they may develop a hypervigilance in carrying out their management roles and become overly suspicious, always looking for possible signs of diversion or intoxication. They may try to relieve their own discomfort by aiming their anger at the impaired professional and may become unreasonably punitive, vindictive, and blaming. They may resent it that someone else wasn't aware or was aware but didn't tell them sooner.

Clearly, this situation can interfere with their ability to perform their work adequately and may estrange the staff they supervise. Certainly, other staff will think twice before telling such a person about other colleagues in trouble, since staff tend to hide information from people who can't handle it. Once this happens, the atmosphere can become very tense, even unhealthy. Management personnel, then, need special reassurance, support, and alleviation of their guilt after the intervention. They can be praised for seeing a problem and addressing it in a courageous and professional way. Never mind that there were some understandable delays. Our blindness and denial are cultural, not simply the fault of people who should have known better.

In one hospital, a superior discovered that a certain nurse had long been diverting Demerol for her own use, then falsifying the records to show that patients had received it. When the superior finally did discover the all-too-obvious falsification of records, she had a hard time forgiving herself for being so "stupid."

Fortunately, she had the good sense to learn from this experience: She developed a policy of completely reviewing all narcotic records at regular intervals. However, managers have so many demands on their time that they simply must delegate certain responsibilities and then trust the delegate unless there are good reasons not to. Until doubts arise, the burden of performance rests on the delegate.

Meeting with Co-workers

Chemically dependent persons don't become or continue that way in total isolation. A collection of friends, family members, and co-workers usually serve as enablers. Most professionals function within systems that put them in touch with many others and possibly with many different disciplines. Even in a limited office practice a physician, dentist, or nurse practitioner interacts with other healthcare professionals on a referral basis, in consultation, or with hospital personnel while making rounds. The same kind of situation is true of law firms. So when impaired professionals are identified, they leave behind an assortment of others who are part of their work environment and who also suffer the impact of intervention, although they often remain invisible to the intervention team.

Chemically dependent professionals affect all those with whom they interact, at least to some degree. On a behavioral level through miscommunication, missed deadlines, temper outbursts and other inappropriate behavior, frequent tardiness, absenteeism, or unrealistic demands, they usually create an increasingly chaotic environment around them. On a practice level, they affect their colleagues through memory lapses, lack of proper follow-through on procedures, inadequate or illegible documentation, errors in judgment, and failure to meet obligations to clients or patients.

This growing inability to meet practice standards usually leads to enabling that prolongs the identification process. Co-workers often "help" the impaired professional by completing work assignments, explaining away unreturned messages, correcting mistakes, and generally making excuses for substandard performance. Over time, enabling is a costly venture, and group productivity decreases. Colleagues, after all, have their own work to do. Emotionally as well, this enabling drains the energy of co-workers as they constantly anticipate their colleague's inability to meet professional responsibilities and as they provide support through the current personal crisis. In fact, there usually are many crises. What isn't evident to many colleagues is that chemical dependence is at the root of the disruption.

Enablers develop their habits slowly and without knowing they're doing anything but giving help. By the time something finally launches the data-collection process, they're firmly entrenched in well-developed enabling roles. When we remove the impaired professional from this web, we find left behind a dysfunctional extended family of co-workers. Roles have been developed around this person who is now gone, at least for a while. That creates confusion and disorganization far beyond the adjustments needed whenever any co-worker is unexpectedly ill and work loads must be adjusted. This work group will also need attention after the intervention.

Before any meetings with the subject's work group, you must of course obtain an appropriate release of information from the subject. You must decide if and when this should occur; it will depend on the particular setting and circumstances. Some subjects give permission at the time of intervention; others may need one to two weeks in treatment before feeling comfortable about having anyone know anything about their problem. This release should specifically name the subject's group and should state simply that the person named may, for the purposes of clarification of feelings and education, discuss the subject's admission to treatment. This release should be witnessed by two persons, and copies should be given to the subject, the intervention coordinator, and the facilitator of any group sessions that will be conducted with co-workers. This is done as soon as possible to provide closure for the work group and to dispel rumors, which by now are usually everywhere in the organization.

We've found that dealing with these situations in groups is extremely effective, whether it be a small office group, the members of a law firm, or an entire nursing staff on a unit. You'll need to consult with the manager of the unit, a senior partner, or the director of an agency to schedule these sessions so that all concerned may attend. Dealing with individual shift groups in hospital units is usually the easiest way to ensure such an opportunity; the offgoing shift stays to cover the unit. People who work closely together are more likely to feel free to express their feelings than they do in a group they don't know very well.

Here are some general guidelines for meeting with co-workers:

1. State the goal of the meeting.
2. Give the group a brief account of the chemically dependent person's status.
3. Provide some general information about chemical dependence in your professional group: attorneys, social workers, healthcare professionals, or whatever the discipline may be.
4. Clarify what happened with the impaired professional.
5. Open the session to the group for response, and listen well.
6. Acknowledge feelings that those present might experience (anger, outrage, guilt, shock, resentment, a sense of failure at not having helped their colleague).
7. Encourage group members to express their feelings, and support them by positive verbal feedback and by physical comforting such as an arm around the shoulder.
8. Conclude the meeting.

Even in very large groups this process is remarkably intense. What one person shares on a personal level is acknowledged by many others who are feeling the same thing but are afraid to be the first to admit how they have felt or are now feeling.

In preparing to deal with the work groups in one inpatient hospital setting, it was decided to divide the groups into their usual work shifts, overlapping shifts attending when possible (one shift coming in a little early). In each meeting there were 25 to 30 co-workers of the absent professional, a nurse who had worked in several units and was well known and well liked. It was determined that the meetings would be open to the other units as well. During one session, several people were crying or near tears. Some were questioning, some denying, and a few clearly angry. These co-workers were able to say openly what they felt and to work through the situation as a group. Each of them had been uniquely affected by this one nurse and needed to be acknowledged, if only by being included in this meeting. As a result, many co-workers wrote letters of support to the nurse in treatment and continued to examine their feelings and share information about chemical dependence with one another.

If these co-workers hadn't been at this meeting, they could easily have had distorted perceptions of what had happened or might mistakenly believe their colleague had simply been fired, perhaps unjustly, for stealing drugs. Always keep in mind that many professionals lack any formal training in chemical dependence and may still view it as a moral or even criminal issue, just as much of society does. Each time an impaired colleague is identified there's a unique opportunity to educate the people involved. This often changes their perspective on the disease and gives them the tools to identify others, sometimes even themselves, much earlier.

In far too many cases people have been removed from the work setting, arrested, or fired without any clarification provided to their co-workers. Those co-workers may never know the truth and can only speculate. They often harbor many feelings of resentment and anger both toward other staff and toward the person in trouble. These negative feelings are damaging to the impaired colleague, to the co-workers, and to the morale of the whole institution. To think that such events can be kept entirely secret is unrealistic. The question isn't whether other people will know, but whether they'll know the truth or settle for gossip and misinformation.

Insofar as you can, then, secure the appropriate releases and then tell the truth, even though you needn't reveal every detail.

If the plan is for the person who's now in treatment to return to the same work site when well enough to do so, you should prepare the groundwork. If "reasonable accommodation to a disability" means modifying the role of the professional in recovery, prepare co-workers for the change. People have been known to return to work situations in which no one knew what had gone wrong, what had happened as a result, what to expect, and who was to keep an eye on the situation to make sure there would be no recurrence of the problem or take steps if there was. Sometimes a person who has returned to work after treatment has had to endure weeks and months of guarded looks, whispers, and suspicion and has had no way of knowing who knows or what they know. Some subjects have been specifically asked by supervisors not to discuss what has happened; this is a great disservice both to the professional in recovery and to co-workers. The result is rumor, conjecture, resentment, and discomfort. If, for example, other nurses are asked to give out medications for a colleague who for a set time isn't allowed to do so, some explanation is in order. Concerns of confidentiality and the demands of reality must be melded with common sense.

In a lecture series on chemical dependence in the healthcare professions at a college of nursing, one of the presenters was an alcoholic professional woman. Her road to recovery had been through the back door in that she had been fired, later arrested twice, and had lost her license before she was finally directed to chemical dependence treatment. At the time of this speaking engagement she had been in recovery a year and a half and had been lecturing frequently on her experiences.

When the audience arrived, she recognized several nurses and other staff with whom she had worked in the hospital that had fired her. She hadn't seen any of them since then and was extremely anxious about their response to her. As she was speaking about her own painful struggle with alcohol/other drugs, particularly in relation to her identification and subsequent termination from the hospital, one of her former co-workers stood up and announced that she had had no idea what had really happened and that all she knew was that the narcotic records were tampered with and names had been forged. She said she had asked questions of her head nurse, but no one would explain or tell her anything. She obviously was still angry and resentful toward everyone involved, although it had happened two years earlier.

The present scene was plainly upsetting to the lecturer (the professional in recovery), so the presiding official (who knew the details of the firing and was an expert on chemical dependence in the workplace) went to the front of the lecture hall and explained what had really happened. The official addressed both the co-worker's anger at the earlier secrecy and at the unprofessional behavior of the administrators and also the underlying guilt that the co-worker was feeling but not mentioning. After the lecture, the co-workers had a chance to talk with the professional in recovery, ask more questions, and express their admiration for her courage in using her negative experience to help others.

The Family of the Impaired Professional

Generally, as we stated earlier, we don't involve family members in an intervention on professionals. We focus on practice-related issues and form a team of professionals and other co-workers to participate in the intervention. However, someone will undoubtedly have to deal with the family either at the time of intervention or immediately afterward.

Remember that the principles of confidentiality say that without a release of information from the subject we have no right to disclose anything to anyone other than the licensing board and the receiving center—not even to the person's family. However, the subject may sometimes ask you to talk to a husband, wife, lover, mother, father, or other significant person to explain the reason for inpatient evaluation or treatment or simply to inform someone that the subject will be going to this facility today.

When possible, it's best if the subject speaks with family members in person, at least by telephone, either before leaving the intervention site or from the treatment center. We generally recommend that the subject tell the family that because of some problems at work, he or she has been requested to be evaluated at the treatment center and that this will involve a few days away. If the family lives nearby, we encourage the subject to have them pack a small overnight bag for the subject and meet him or her at the treatment center. This serves two purposes. First, it avoids having the impaired professional take detours on the way to the facility; second, it provides the treatment staff with the opportunity to meet with the family, provide them support, and begin the necessary information-gathering from them (family assessment). Rather than get involved in lengthy explanations on the phone, the subject is encouraged to let the family know that an explanation will come later.

Sometimes the subject may ask the coordinator or a team member who knows the family to phone and ask them to come to the hospital or office and pick up the subject. In this case, the subject is usually seated with the person doing the phoning, and the family is told the subject isn't feeling well and has asked that they be called. When the family arrives, the subject will usually sum up what has happened and look for their support. This is also an opportunity for the intervention team to show concern and demonstrate they still care and have no intention of rejecting the person.

Of course not all families are going to respond with approval and gratitude; there are always those who defy anyone to do or say anything about one of their own. Be prepared for hostile phone calls, spouses who make threats, people indignant that anyone can think their son, daughter, wife, husband, or lover is using alcohol/other drugs. These confrontations may occur even in your office and can be quite unpleasant. But remember, you're dealing with people who themselves are caught up in the situation—enablers who are afraid for themselves and have something to lose. The impaired professional is often the financial backbone of the family, and his or her removal from the work force is often a serious threat to the family's economic well-being. No wonder intervention causes a reaction from spouse, family members, and significant others.

In dealing with these people, then, you must be calm, never defensive. When speaking with families, choose your words carefully; don't label the subject as chemically dependent, and don't volunteer your personal impressions as to the cause of the problem. It's usually best simply to restate that you're not at liberty to discuss the details of the situation with them; instead, refer them to the treatment counselor. Sometimes, though, you may have to meet promptly with the subject, family, and treatment staff to go over what led up to the intervention and to discuss the likely consequences if there's no treatment. This will usually force the family to accept the situation, since they can't change it. This meeting with the family isn't as urgent when the subject's license or position is on the line as it is when persuasion is practically your only clout. So if you aren't prepared to explain the situation calmly and objectively, the family can easily destroy everything you've done, not because they're malicious, but from lack of knowledge and hence fear.

Taking Care of Yourself

Now that you've taken care of the intervention team, the subject, the facility managers, the work group, and the family, you have another task: taking care of yourself. As professionals, we're used to giving of ourselves physically and emotionally, but dealing with chemical dependence is especially demanding emotionally in that it requires endless patience, the ability to care about people who seemingly don't care about themselves, and persistence in facing people who flatly deny the existence of the problem—not only those who have it, but those involved with those who have it! Quite a tall order for one lonely intervention coordinator, particularly one who's new to the whole procedure and in fact is quite unused to handling problems of this kind! Good for you that you cared enough and had enough courage to do it!

Each of us has the right and responsibility to restore our own inner selves, not only in order to maintain our effectiveness, but also to hang on to a degree of personal peace. We can't consistently meet the needs of others without meeting our own. To spend all of our earned interest is fine, but we must be wary of borrowing from capital. We each meet our needs differently, but we must meet them. Without conscious attention to this final task, you may find yourself drained and unable to detach from the intervention process, particularly if you do interventions frequently. We didn't go through all this work to deal with someone else's impairment only to set the stage for developing problems of our own. Here are some suggestions:

1. Arrange to meet with a good confidant and talk out your feelings about the intervention. (If you have no such person, **think** about that.)
2. Attend or join a 12-Step program such as Al-Anon. (For those continually involved with chemical dependents, either in personal relationships or in intervention, we recommend regular attendance.)
3. Reduce your distractions and stress for a while. Put on the answering machine, drop the children at a movie or a friend's house, set a specific time for relaxation. Always TV? Why not try music instead? Does everything you do have to be useful or improve something?
4. Take yourself and a good companion to dinner in a special restaurant.
5. Treat yourself to a massage or a manicure. Pamper yourself.
6. Go to the gym or spa. Swim. Move!
7. Plan a weekend getaway—and actually go.
8. Get together with the special people in your life.
9. Congratulate yourself for caring enough about another person to accept the risk and challenge of intervention.

Chapter Highlights

After intervention, coordinators are responsible for addressing the needs of the intervention team members, co-workers and colleagues of the impaired professional, families of the impaired professional, and their own needs.

Here are the chief needs of the intervention team:
1. Clarification of the events
2. Identification of feelings
3. Expression of feelings
4. Mutual support and reassurance
5. Closure to the intervention

At a meeting with co-workers and colleagues you should:
1. Define goals for the meeting.
2. Provide brief objective information regarding the impaired professional, including what conditions will govern the person's return to work.
3. Discuss chemical dependence.
4. Acknowledge the feelings of those present.
5. Encourage discussion of feelings.
6. Clarify events and feelings for the group.
7. Encourage group interaction and support.
8. Provide closure.

In dealing with families you should:
1. Encourage the impaired person to notify them at the time of intervention.
2. Request them to meet the subject at the evaluation center.
3. Maintain confidentiality.
4. Request assistance from the treatment center in dealing with families who are hostile, angry, and/or threatening.

For suggestions on taking care of yourself, see the list just presented on page 179.

Chapter 8

Phase 4:
Treatment and Recovery

Through your efforts your impaired colleague is off on what we hope will prove to be the road to healing and restoration. Some impaired colleagues, naturally, won't see the intervention and treatment as much of a gift until therapy is well advanced, and some remain angry and resentful for quite a while. They won't be grateful for the great caring and energy we've expended; instead, they feel they've unwillingly been removed from life as they knew it. Everyone around them knows they've been on a progressively destructive course, but their defense system won't let them see it. Understanding and acceptance (as against mere compliance) will come if the treatment plan is followed and there's no return to alcohol/other drugs, but it may take several weeks or months. For now, you must entrust your colleague to the expert care of the evaluation staff at the selected treatment center.

Evaluation

Before evaluation starts, you as coordinator must in many cases take care of the important matter of release forms.

Release-of-Information Forms

Once the impaired professional arrives at the evaluation site, your communications and contacts will be with the counselors there. Counselors may be of different professional disciplines. If you play a formal role in the evaluation and treatment process, you must first provide the center with a written release from the impaired professional stating that you have his or her permission to discuss pertinent facts with the counselors. Then you may contact the treating professionals and relay information, facts, events that may significantly help in their evaluation. However, they may not share, discuss, or acknowledge any information without a separate release form from the impaired professional that clearly states that they may discuss relevant information with you or other designated individuals. Until this release is signed, the counselors may not even acknowledge the presence of the professional in their facility. Persons being treated in chemical dependence hospitals and centers are protected under federal confidentiality laws, and most centers take this quite seriously.

Confidentiality must be rigidly observed, as we've learned by experience. One of us was formerly closely connected to a treatment center where celebrities were often among our patients. No one was admitted there except for suspected or verified chemical dependence, so presence alone implied the diagnosis. Reporters and even curious casual acquaintances would call frequently, pretending to know that someone was there, "just to ask how Joe's doing," or with a seemingly innocent request to pass along a message. The response had to be, "Even if such a person were here I wouldn't be at liberty to tell you." Patients need and appreciate the care taken to protect their privacy. In some places, alcoholism and other drug addictions still carry stigma, and we must acknowledge that.

The Evaluation Itself

Some chemical dependence centers with experience in treating impaired professionals offer a four-day evaluation program using certain members of the treatment team, a physician with expertise in addiction to alcohol/other drugs, a psychiatrist, a psychologist, and chemical dependence counselors. The work of this team includes family and social assessments, history, review of the subject's alcohol/other drug use, medical and psychiatric evaluation, and review and interpretation of the data submitted by the intervention team. At the end of the evaluation process, the treatment team meets to formulate its conclusions and to make its recommendations. These recommendations are shared with the subject and other appropriate persons (peer assistance, employer, licensing board) designated on the release forms.

These final recommendations present the impaired professional with objective reality, usually saying that the person does need chemical dependence treatment. It has been our experience, and that of many colleagues in the field, that almost all professionals do comply, at least initially, with the recommended treatment if the intervention has been planned well and carried out well. They know the consequences of failure to comply. Many subjects are essentially in a no-win situation, expressed aptly by a pharmacist who said after intervention, "You're giving me two choices, but there's really no choice." That's precisely what leverage in effective intervention with impaired professionals is all about! The choice the subject would like, of deciding that things are really just fine and that everything can now go on just as before, really isn't available.

If you hold a position within the peer assistance program or are the professional's employer, you may be invited, with the permission of the impaired professional, to attend the evaluation summary meeting at the treatment center. The purpose of your attendance is multiple: 1) You hold some type of leverage over the subject, such as continued employment or practice; 2) you can initiate a second intervention at the treatment center if the subject rejects treatment; 3) your presence reinforces to the subject your continued support and encouragement, which can alleviate anxiety and fear about the subject's continued professional practice; and 4) you and the treatment team can establish that you're working together on the patient's behalf. It's not a good-guy-versus-bad-guy situation.

Treatment

Many impaired professionals feel that by submitting to chemical dependence treatment they'll be publicly acknowledging their weakness, and they feel particularly vulnerable to professional and collegial criticism. The ongoing support of another significant professional figure makes clear, however, that someone within the profession accepts them despite their difficulties, even though that colleague insists that they make a major investment in getting well. This expression of continued care and concern is crucial and provides considerable reassurance in a situation they perceive as gloomy at best.

If the professional is evaluated at a center outside your area, you may request (using a release form signed at the time of intervention) a formal written summary of its findings and recommendations. Since you've already asked the subject not only to be evaluated but also to comply with the recommendations that follow, you must be sure this happens, particularly when noncompliance may mean that you'll initiate disciplinary or suspension procedures to protect the public. It's advisable that you request not only a written summary but also phone notification from the evaluating center at the completion of the evaluation meeting. When a professional has been identified as impaired and unable to meet the standards of practice, we clearly have an ethical obligation to ensure that recommendations will be followed. Treatment is a process, not an outcome. It's by no means enough for people to complete it and appear well; we must make sure they stay well. Usually that means at least two years of monitoring after inpatient treatment before we can conclude that the person has achieved a stable sobriety and understands the need for lifelong abstinence plus involvement in an ongoing recovery program such as A.A. or N.A. Relapse can occur in most illnesses, and chemical dependence is no exception. In our experience, most impaired professionals who are chemically dependent receive a minimum of 28 days of inpatient treatment; the discussions that follow in this chapter assume this type of treatment. (For descriptions of current forms of treatment, see Appendix A.)

Some professionals do recover with no treatment at all beyond what they find in mutual-support groups such as Alcoholics Anonymous. However, when you've identified signs of impaired practice and have had to force the issue of treatment, relying solely on such groups would be too little, too late. You accepted the responsibility for finding the resources most likely to lead to successful recovery, and that means formal treatment by experts. If anything, it's probably better to overtreat than to gamble on what may not be enough.

Progress Reports

If you're accountable for documenting the treatment and progress of the chemically dependent professional, you'll need to establish your expectations of the treatment center early on. Some centers have well-defined protocols for weekly progress reports (and, of course, appropriate release forms) issued routinely to persons responsible for the impaired professional. If the center is local, you may even receive weekly calls from the primary counselor reporting the progress of the impaired professional and, in general terms, specifying areas in which difficulties remain. The information disclosed isn't usually intimate or detailed but deals rather with broader issues that affect progress toward rehabilitation as a trustworthy professional. Since the patient has a right to privacy, the details of family interactions, unrelated physical problems, romantic entanglements, sexual orientation, religious views, and the like are none of our business.

Inpatient Interventions

If the professional is demonstrating significant resistance to treatment, the counselor may ask you to participate in a second intervention at the treatment center. Usually this occurs early in treatment, when subjects are experiencing painful emotional withdrawal from alcohol/other drugs and therefore are more vehement than ever in denying that they need any treatment at all.

Additionally, they may attempt to dissociate themselves from the other patients by saying, "I don't belong here" or "These are laymen; I'm a doctor" or "I have nothing in common with these people; half of them are addicts and the other half are drunks." Professionals try to use "I'm a skilled surgeon," "I'm a nun," "I'm a psychologist," "I'm a congressman" to avoid looking at other chemically dependent professionals as basically like themselves. They'd rather emphasize the difference: "I'm not like **these** people." We hear the same sort of words from the patients at Guest House, a facility for Catholic priests; each of them feels that what applies to the other priests, nice though they are, and much though they might need help, doesn't apply to him. This attitude isn't automatically overcome by putting members of the same occupational group together, though it helps not to be the only doctor, nun, or lawyer in the place.

To help the treatment team you should prepare copies of the data shared in the original intervention and review for yourself the leverage you have to convince the impaired professional that staying in treatment is the best option. On the designated day you'll meet with the treatment team immediately before the intervention and be briefed on how the meeting will proceed. They now have their own documentation to present, new data about what they know of the impaired professional. Such data has great impact.

When the impaired professional arrives, the treatment team leader will tell the subject the purpose of the meeting and will ask the subject not to speak until asked to. The intervention now is very much like the one you completed some days or weeks ago, except for one important factor: The chemical dependence has now been diagnosed. Now it can be named and addressed directly and candidly by the treatment team. It's very difficult for the subject to intimidate or deceive this treatment team, since the members have great expertise in dealing with chemically dependent people. That, combined with the documentation you've summarized, really gives the professional no choice but to agree at least to go through the motions without wasting energy trying to escape treatment.

Your role should be that of a concerned colleague offering continued support to the subject who agrees to work through the treatment program. Depending on the subject's emotional state, he or she may not acknowledge your commitment to be truly helpful, but be assured it doesn't go unnoticed. We remember completing a second intervention on a nurse after the first week of treatment and attempting to offer a gesture of support by placing an arm around her shoulder. The nurse remained unresponsive and walked away. But when the nurse's treatment was completed she acknowledged that on that day she had felt so hopeless she couldn't really respond to much of anything. But she distinctly remembered the arm around her shoulder and the feeling that she wasn't alone—that someone had reached out to her even though she was acting miserably toward everyone involved. In short, recovering professionals sharing their memories of intervention remember very clearly who reached out to comfort and reassure them in their distress.

Long-Term Treatment Recommendations

By the third or fourth week of treatment, the treatment team will meet and share observations, concerns, and recommendations. If long-term treatment is indicated, it will be presented to the subject at a meeting held early in the final week. Again, you may be present if the position you hold qualifies you as needing to know and if the proper releases have been signed. Recommendations for more treatment may meet the same objections you heard at intervention: "This isn't fair. I did what you said, and now you say it's not enough," "I can't go; I have things to take care of" (children, pets, finances), "I can't afford it; I have no more money," and so forth. If subjects need more treatment it's usually because they're still minimizing or denying reality and haven't faced up to their problem enough to have much chance of recovering. At this point the treatment team will explain its perspective and reasoning, while you may summarize and reemphasize for the professional the performance issues that led to treatment in the first place. This is really almost another mini intervention to help professional subjects see that although they've made progress, they're not yet well and need further treatment. Again, if resistance and denial persist, you can still use your leverage of disciplinary action but in a factual, nonthreatening way. "Mary, when we intervened you agreed to follow the recommendations of the team here at the center. They think you need continued treatment. Our agreement was that if you didn't follow the recommendations made, I'd have to report to the bar what happened and say that you refused to comply with what the treatment team has proposed. Before you came here to treatment, Mary, your clients were unsafe because of your chemical dependence, and I can't allow you to return to the courtroom with treatment unfinished."

As we explained earlier, the impaired professional often attempts to bargain. "Couldn't I just go home and come to aftercare twice a week instead of once?" or "I'll take a different job" or "I could stay away from taking on new clients for a few months while I get counseling." Professionals some-times do successfully manipulate acceptance of their own treatment plans—and if they do, usually fail to get well. But most professionals referred to extended treatment after the initial four-week treatment do eventually agree to further treatment. Their foot-dragging isn't evidence of bad faith. Since people in inpatient treatment are removed from the environmental cues that tempt them to drink or use and usually experience very little craving while there, the safe surroundings can create a false sense of security. Many have no awareness of how difficult a sustained recovery can be.

Preparing for the Discharge

About the third week of a 28-day program the treatment staff assesses the progress of the subject and explores what further formal treatment is indi-cated. If there's not to be a transfer to extended care, the staff will develop a discharge plan for the professional, and if an extended-care facility is involved, that staff will complete discharge planning at the appropriate time.

If you've participated in the evaluation, treatment, and progress confer-ences, you'll of course be included in the discharge planning. You may need to make sure the treatment team understands any requirements the impaired professional must meet as employee, as peer assistance participant, or as subject to the rules of any other program, so that the discharge plans are cohesive and inclusive. Your criteria may be relayed to the counselor by phone, but it's advisable to send a written statement as well. Most counselors will incorporate all the pertinent criteria into a comprehensive plan for the recovering professional.

A basic aftercare or discharge plan will include:
1. Specific outpatient therapy or counseling, how often and with whom
2. Aftercare and other meetings, how often per week (days and times)
3. Number of 12-Step program meetings per week (which specific pro-grams)
4. Recommended work hours
5. Restrictions on practice
6. Abstinence from all mind-altering drugs
7. Methods by which abstinence will be monitored, such as urine screens (by whom) and permission to do so
8. Professional support group attendance (how often)
9. Obtaining a sponsor in a 12-Step program (what date)

10. Participation in professional peer assistance programs
11. Other recommendations as appropriate

These plans are usually typed in the form of agreements to be signed by both the primary counselor and the recovering person at a formal discharge conference.

While the treatment team is developing its discharge plan, you need to prepare your own guidelines for the professional in recovery if you represent either a peer assistance or impairment program or the professional's primary employer. The general framework of your planning for the professional's discharge will be based on the type of role you've assumed and the projected recommendations of the treatment team about return to practice. You and the primary counselor should get together before the formal discharge conference so that the expectations on both sides are clear and are presented without contradictions to the professional in recovery.

Roles You May Play in Discharge Planning

1. The Peer Assistance Role. If you're a peer assistance representative, your program will provide written guidelines for the professional's participation in the program. The guidelines may include such items as these: 1) an overall agreement that the subject will follow the guidelines for a specific time; 2) specific expectations of the treatment discharge plan; 3) methods of monitoring recovery (urine testing and progress reports required); 4) an agreement to have two sponsors (one person from a 12-Step group, one from a professional recovery group); 5) abstinence from mind-altering chemicals; 6) restrictions on practice; 7) how relapse will be dealt with; and 8) general statements about the consequences of noncompliance with the formal agreement. The specific issues addressed may differ slightly in each program; these are only samples of the general areas covered in peer assistance agreements. (Appendices B and C have examples of such agreements.)

As a representative you'll need to prepare for the professional in recovery an agreement based on the requirements of the program, recommendations of the treatment team, and other particular needs of the individual professional. A major consideration is the professional's ability to practice when discharged. If your program philosophy is that all such professionals must remain inactive for a time, this must be shared with the treatment team upon admission so that the team may help the professional to accept this gradually, rather than waiting to deliver the blow on the day of discharge. Despite the fact that you may yourself have explained this to the professional early in treatment, the subject may have been unable to hear the message and may have hoped that if he or she does well in treatment you might relent. The primary counselor must know your policy and may present it again at a point in treatment when the professional is able to listen.

If your program doesn't have a rigid nonpractice philosophy, are there nevertheless restrictions to practice? In many programs for healthcare professionals, limitations are imposed on handling of medications for a time. This policy has weighty implications for professionals whose practice requires administration of these substances: physician assistants, anesthesiologists, pharmacists, veterinarians, and nurses, for example. If any other restrictions exist, they too must be shared with the treatment counselors as they prepare the professional for discharge. Will the professional be limited to "supervised practice"? If so, this has a critical impact on the recovering professional's scope of practice and may severely limit the practice setting as well.

If the program doesn't have standard recommendations for practice by professionals in early recovery, does the treatment team itself have recommendations regarding practice limitations? If so, you must include these in the individualized plan for the professional after discussing them with the primary counselor. Planning for the professional's discharge when there are limitations of practice is critical. The lists of expectations suddenly placed before the professional may be overwhelming, and the person may be able to focus only on the subject of practice. Initially the primary response may be "How will I ever find another job?" or "They won't want me back if I can't give medications" or "Who's going to hire a drug addict?" or "I don't know how to do anything else" or "I'm in debt up to my ears; how will I survive?" You can support and encourage by sharing stories of other program participants and the ways in which they were able to continue practice. Also, it's advisable that you make concrete suggestions to professionals about names of agencies and types of employment in which they can use their skills while still adhering to program requirements. Some peer assistance programs, through their demonstrated success, have many resources for employment of their participants, and some of these may be shared with professionals after discharge. Some colleagues who work in peer assistance programs joke that they do as much job placement as they do intervention!

You may want to send the professional a copy of the completed tentative contract to review during the third week or so of treatment (or while the person is in long-term treatment). This gives the subject an opportunity to study it, discuss it with counselors and colleagues, and bring up any significant concerns or questions with you before final agreement at the time of discharge.

If you're geographically close and have the time to meet with the professional, you may request this meeting through the primary counselor.

This is ideal, because it's much more effective to communicate in person and work out details. We've learned through experience that a hidden benefit of this personal touch is that the professional has usually undergone a significant physical recovery and looks like quite a different person. In some cases, this change is dramatic and visually confirms why our intervention was needed; besides, it lets the professional know how wonderful he or she looks. This positive feedback is very meaningful, particularly from someone who saw the person at his or her worst. To show the physical changes of recovery, many centers take Polaroid photos of the person at the time of admission and at discharge and let the patient see the difference.

2. The Employer's Role. If you're the primary employer of the recovering professional, your planning for after the discharge will depend on several factors: 1) treatment-team recommendations for employment or practice; 2) guidelines of the peer assistance program (if one exists); 3) your institution's policy regarding professionals in recovery; and 4) your commitment to providing alternatives for using the expertise and skills of the professional while adhering to any required limitations of practice. This is obviously more tricky for healthcare workers than for clergy, attorneys, psychologists, social workers, or teachers.

Clearly, as employer you've already demonstrated your support of the professional by the intervention itself and by your subsequent communications with the counselors. In anticipating the professional's discharge, your foremost concern is of course the person's ability to return to practice. This decision will be shared with the treatment team in collaboration with any peer assistance program within the state. You may already know, by working with your state programs, of general practice restrictions for all recovering professionals that limit what you can offer, and you can explore alternatives within your agency or institution early in the treatment process. The healthcare professions often limit practice simply to prevent access to drugs. Many programs for nurses, doctors, pharmacists, and veterinarians state that the professional in recovery may not handle or prescribe narcotics or other potentially addictive drugs for six months to a year. Initially an employer's response may be, "I can't have a nurse who can't give drugs. It's not fair to burden the others" or "He can't go back to intensive care without being able to give drugs." These are very common responses from employers who haven't fully explored alternatives for placing the recovering professional in areas of practice that will benefit both the employer and the professional.

A nurse anesthetist who was chemically dependent and had diverted large quantities of Fentanyl (a synthetic narcotic) was identified and intervened with by the hospital. He subsequently completed a four-week treatment program and on the recommendation of his counselors was cleared to return to work with the provision that he adhere to the state program's guidelines of "no administration or handling of narcotics." His department head didn't want to lose a very talented practitioner and therefore created a position for a clinical nurse anesthetist educator in the operating room. Actual instruction and training was conducted outside the operating room itself, which remained off limits as agreed upon. He quickly assumed other special projects in addition to education and was a valuable asset to the department.

Another case was that of an experienced intensive-care nurse who after inpatient chemical dependence treatment was cleared to return to work with similar restrictions: no handling of narcotics. This nurse had ten years of clinical experience in critical care and was well liked by her co-workers, who were very supportive during her treatment. The hospital was reluctant to place her back in the intensive-care unit in view of the restrictions imposed by the state program. Its position was that each nurse in intensive care assumed total responsibility for each patient, including all required medications. With the nurse's permission, a meeting was held with the staff in the intensive-care unit, the supervisor, and the peer assistance advocate to discuss the feasibility of the nurse's returning to work under those restrictions. Her co-workers quickly resolved the problem by stating that each day someone would be assigned to administer medications to her patients and that in turn she would assume responsibility for treatments for one of the assigned nurse's patients. When she did return to work, the system worked quite well and served as an excellent example of what could be done.

Of course, not all professionals can return to their prior professional practice roles, and this presents a more difficult problem for employers. For some reason, employers are slow to offer positions to professionals that don't actually require their credentials. Agencies or facilities, depending upon their size, may have a variety of nonclinical positions they could offer professionals in recovery but are sometimes reluctant to do so, perhaps for fear of insulting them. But there's no reason why nurses, pharmacists, and even physicians, for example, can't assume new roles within the organization when they're ready to return to work. Hospitals may consider positions in central supply, admitting, quality review, discharge planning, infectious disease, physical therapy, and employee health as feasible for the professional who may not return immediately to full clinical practice. The obvious advantage of expending your energies in placing this person is that you're retaining a valuable employee and also providing support and encouragement during the recovery process.

Don't forget to ask for suggestions from the peer assistance program and/ or the treatment staff in considering possible areas of employment. Nurses in recovery, for example, have gained employment in department stores, florist shops, post offices, and various other work positions as they worked through the initial stages of their recovery. Pharmacists have taught science.

Once you've determined the feasibility of the professional's returning to the workplace, you should discuss these options with the primary counselor before the discharge meeting. The counselor may wish to discuss these options with the professional in advance so that a definite plan may be presented at the discharge meeting. In the meantime, you can be preparing for possible job placement and begin developing your own return-to-work contract to be ready before the professional's first day back at work.

It's recommended that you attend the discharge planning meeting at the treatment center to hear firsthand the treatment recommendations, peer assistance and other requirements for the professional in recovery, and to receive written copies of both. If you can't attend, request copies of the material presented through the primary counselor. It's imperative that you have specific knowledge of these contracts, since they should serve as the foundation of the contract you'll be designing.

Recovery Issues

In discussing recovery, one of the first issues we need to consider is ongoing treatment in the form of aftercare.

Aftercare

Aftercare is the less-intensive phase of treatment that continues, usually for one to two years, after a person is discharged from an inpatient treatment program. It usually consists of weekly or biweekly formal support groups facilitated by the treatment center staff. It's a way for the subject to reinforce and practice the new behaviors and lifeskills acquired in treatment while receiving feedback on progress from colleagues. It's one more step in the process of recovery. The person now begins to reexperience life in the real world and relies heavily on support from 12-Step programs, professional support groups, aftercare, and all the activities the personal recovery plan provides. Professionals in recovery can be extremely busy people, always seeming to be running to a meeting or group. They are. Certainly one objective is to minimize the time left unstructured and to keep their efforts focused on their recovery. In planning for this early recovery phase, peer assistance programs and employers can smooth the transition by doing careful discharge planning, offering the subject sensible employment options, and sending the subject any required contracts well ahead of time so that the subject can have time to inspect the requirements for participation in the impaired-professional program before signing the contracts. If possible, those sharing responsibility for the person should keep in touch with one another and not simply assume that everything is going as planned.

Aftercare is a most important part of the treatment process. Upon discharge, professionals are just beginning the work of dealing with their chemical dependence. As they leave the protection of the treatment center, life with all its problems and temptations is waiting. Granted, they've gained a new perspective on living and may look forward to homecoming, but they'll undoubtedly face great stress as they pick up the pieces.

The primary counselor assigns the professional to a specific aftercare group that meets on set days and times in order to provide group stability and trust. The subject may also be assigned a new counselor, hereafter referred to as the aftercare counselor. You, as a person of influence, help employers and other schedule makers to understand that people new in recovery need to attend these sessions in order to stay well and to fulfill their obligation to follow through with treatment. Such people should not be hampered by last-minute requests to stay late or work extra shifts if that interferes with their attendance. For some, returning home isn't easy, and even though their families may have participated in the program at the center, many changes lie ahead for all of them. Renewing contact with friends, assuming responsibility for finances, or attempting to secure a new job if the old one has been lost or the license removed can rock the boat of recovery for those who are still learning about themselves and about what recovery is like outside the treatment center. Regular attendance at aftercare answers their continued need for feedback, redirection, and encouragement.

The aftercare counselor may also provide progress reports and periodic updates to responsible persons (such as peer assistance coordinators, employers, or directors of regulatory programs) and in some cases is responsible for submitting formal documentation of attendance and compliance with recommendations to regulatory (impairment) programs. Aftercare recommendations are specifically delineated in the discharge plan (see the previous section, Preparing for the Discharge). Noncompliance with this continued treatment should be confronted promptly and taken quite seriously. Professionals in recovery sometimes start missing meetings with or without an excuse—behavior that should be addressed at once by the aftercare counselor, who reminds the person of the agreement signed. When this behavior persists, the counselor will usually notify the person who monitors the professional's ongoing treatment. Then that person, perhaps in conjunction with the after-care counselor, will meet with the professional in recovery to spell out yet again that he or she is expected to comply with all recommended treatment. As the person progresses in recovery, the attendance requirements for aftercare may change and a new agreement may be made. For example, in early recovery, say for the first six months, aftercare groups may meet two or three times weekly, then with satisfactory progress only once or twice weekly. Of course each program is different, and requirements will vary, depending on individuals, specific stipulations of any formal impairment program they're participating in, and the philosophy of the treatment center.

One of the most frustrating problems you'll face is to have a person do very well in inpatient treatment but then have to remain in extended residential treatment because no decent aftercare is available nearby. Sometimes people who could recover perfectly well with good aftercare make several false starts and even fail altogether because they simply can't drive or fly hundreds of miles to where it's available. You may have to settle for intensive weekend programs provided by many excellent treatment centers available throughout the country, or for residential refreshers or similar stopgaps in addition to the mutual-support groups.

But don't write anyone off. Self-help groups for chemical dependents are meeting by computer and by ham radio and a variety of other systems, but all concerned may have to use a lot of ingenuity. One woman religious, a nursing sister on a remote Indian reservation, managed quite well with telephone contacts alone, although we don't consider this an adequate form of aftercare.

Progress Reports

Although release forms were obtained during the inpatient treatment phase, new releases must be signed when there's any change of counselors. In the aftercare phase of treatment the professional in recovery will most likely have a new counselor. This counselor will then be a primary contact for whoever is responsible for monitoring the progress of the professional, and the release will specifically give you permission to receive information from this person.

When these releases are completed, you should initiate contact with the professional's new aftercare counselor by phone and request periodic progress reports in writing. These reports, as with all documentation related to the professional, should be secured in a nonaccessible locked file. Establish your position with the treatment center so that a discharge plan is sent to you a little before the person is actually discharged. Make clear that delays in sending needed records, usually blamed on dictating and slow transcribing, are simply not going to be acceptable and that if the facility can't provide these documents, you'll have to refer elsewhere in future. You may have to be firm about this, but even the best treatment centers must compete for patients, and most are eager to have professionals as patients.

Return-to-Work Contracts

If you're an employer of professionals in recovery, you're strongly urged to prepare a contract that spells out the expectations that they must meet as a condition of continued employment. It should include statements related to:

1. Compliance with all treatment recommendations as detailed in the discharge plan
2. Compliance with peer assistance and state program guidelines
3. Abstinence from all mind-altering substances
4. Agreement to submit to random blood or urine samples on request, and to be tested for presence of these substances
5. Agreement to participate in any existing recovery programs sponsored by the employer, such as support groups for professionals in recovery
6. Agreement not to use any prescribed medications without approval of a designated individual physician who's knowledgeable about chemical dependence or who will first consult with a designated one who is
7. Permission to the employer or a specific designee to communicate with the person's primary treatment counselor (specific person) to discuss or document the person's ongoing recovery, and an understanding that any relapse unreported (either by the professional, counselor, or peer assistance program) could be grounds for termination

The treatment discharge plan will be quite comprehensive in spelling out suggested meeting attendance, sponsorship, support groups, and therapy; but what you're now establishing in this return-to-work contract is that you, the employer, also maintain responsibility to ensure safe practice with the help of all the steps outlined in the contract. You're not inventing new ones in order to assert yourself or complicate matters. This contract should be discussed in person with the professional in recovery before the person returns to work, not squeezed into the day of the subject's return. In some facilities the contract is developed by a committee composed of representatives of the department in which the person will work, a personnel advisor, or an employee assistance counselor, and with advice from a peer assistance program. This contract should ideally be written in such a way that while it lends itself to individualization, it follows established policy for all professional employees in recovery.

Once a generic contract form is developed, it's advisable to have it reviewed by the attorney(s) who represent the organization. (See samples in Appendix D.) Be prepared for attorneys to know little about chemical dependence, and don't be surprised if their first impulse is to get rid of the person rather than help with a sensible monitoring system. You're probably away ahead of them on this issue. But you can contact similar institutions or employers who have developed very satisfactory contracts and guidelines for returning professionals to the workplace.

Role Modifications/Adaptations in the Workplace

If the professional in recovery is returning to the original employer, several types of stress will predictably result:

1. Stress from new restrictions on professional practice
2. Stress from role changes if assuming a new professional assignment
3. Stress due to perceived or actual hostile or suspicious attitudes on the part of other staff
4. Self-imposed stress caused by trying to make up for past mistakes by being perfect and trying to show how competent he or she is
5. Stress from adjustments with friends and family
6. Stress in meeting all contract obligations while working full-time as well

Awareness of the person's feelings is paramount to assisting him or her through these transitions. Knowing that professionals are generally high achievers (or they wouldn't be where they are) and identifying strongly with their chosen profession prepares us to deal with the feelings of professional inadequacy or failure when an experienced practitioner returns to work but is limited in opportunity to perform. For compulsive, well-organized skillful practitioners it's a humbling experience to have to depend on others to shoulder their responsibilities. Nurses, for instance, have strong feelings about imposing on others to give their medications and often feel particularly inadequate when a patient requests pain medication and they must wait for someone else to give it. They need support, understanding, and encouragement. Eventually, as they discuss these feelings, usually with the support of other colleagues in recovery, they're able to focus on their clinical expertise in other areas such as patient assessment and medical interventions rather than on the restrictions applying to their administration of medications. But adjustment doesn't happen overnight! When the professional in recovery has told co-workers exactly **why** he or she can't give medications, for instance, those co-workers can provide both acceptance and support for the professional.

Assuming a new work role can also be quite stressful. For example, two nurses chose to function as ward clerks in a hospital rather than leave a supportive employer and start over somewhere else. Both these women experienced considerable discomfort, since the change represented a major drop in status. But through their aftercare, other support groups, and caring co-workers they accepted their new roles and developed a new sense of personal competence in having met this challenge and survived. Self-worth doesn't come only through a particular occupation, but that isn't always easy to learn.

Professionals who choose to work in unrelated jobs may experience some anxiety about dropping out of their chosen profession. Most don't want to lose their identity as professionals or lose touch with their colleagues, but some simply need time away from the demands and expectations of their practice. These people may need reassurance that they still belong to their professional group and aren't going to lose their competence or be forgotten even though they've chosen to work elsewhere. Even those who mistakenly blame their profession for causing their chemical dependence usually focus their hostility on a tangible object such as "that hospital," "that counseling clinic," "that supervisor," "that parish," or "that law firm" rather than on the profession as a whole. Always keep in mind how closely many professionals identify with their professional group and how hard they've worked to achieve the privilege of membership! Even social workers working in roles almost unrelated to their original training will often show a special feeling for other social workers.

Work Schedules for Professionals in Recovery

Many treatment programs suggest that the returning professional keep to a "normal" and predictable life schedule in the first few months after treatment. As we discussed earlier, there will be significant demands on the professional's time to attend meetings, counseling, and aftercare; and in most communities (except of course for major metropolitan areas) accessibility to recovery meetings is limited except during the evening hours. Another obvious consideration in setting up work schedules is that we all function on a circadian cycle, which means that our body clocks are programmed for primary alertness during daytime hours, relaxation and winding down during evening hours, and regeneration (sleep) during night hours. Attempting to alter these processes does result in physiological stress. Of course in our society there's a subculture of night people who have managed to adjust to the opposite of this cycle. We often wonder how successfully they've done it, though, when we review the incidence of stress-related illness and job-related injuries or accidents in night workers. We attempt to maintain a normal life balance for persons in recovery by putting them in daytime positions so they can work on their recovery plan, spend quality time with their families and friends, and maintain a normal balance of sleep and rest and other activities. There's also better supervision at work during the day, so if problems arise, they're more likely to be detected then.

The discharge plan may advise that professionals in recovery be limited in the total number of hours they work. The temptation is great to work overtime so as to catch up financially and perhaps also to show gratitude to co-workers and employers by covering when staffing is minimal. This is probably unwise and is decidedly so if staying to cover means missing a treatment session or aftercare group.

Disciplinary/Licensure Issues

Some professionals must face disciplinary proceedings after their discharge from treatment. Unfortunately, not all states have advocacy programs, and it's required that after discharge professionals must be reported to the appropriate boards and receive disciplinary action. This is very painful when the person has complied with all treatment recommendations and is staying off alcohol/ other drugs but still faces a disciplining procedure decided on long after it serves any purpose beyond doling out punishment. However, in many states there's often less severe action when the professional can document successful chemical dependence treatment and continued aftercare. The severity of the action depends on the state and/or the profession involved. It can range from probationary status for a one- to two-year period without loss of full practice privileges to suspension of privilege to practice for a specific time or even to revocation. During these proceedings, it's critical to provide support to professionals newly in recovery and have a colleague accompany them to any formal hearings. Skilled legal advice can be invaluable.

Methods of Monitoring Recovery

Many programs responsible for helping identify impaired professionals also monitor the professional in recovery. Monitoring is a particularly central issue for programs that offer protection from disciplinary action by the licensing boards, bar, credentialing boards, and such. These programs must safeguard the public and ensure that the professional is competent to practice.

Similarly, advocates strive to safeguard professionals in recovery from slander, libel, and false accusations. When they return to their practice or community, their recovery may be questioned. For example, a nurse returning to work in the hospital where her intervention took place was working on a large medical unit. Although by agreement she had no access to narcotics, she was the primary suspect when Demerol was missing from the narcotic cabinet. When she realized that other nurses thought her the most likely suspect, she immediately notified the Director of Nursing and asked to have a urine sample collected for a drug screen. Since this nurse had periodically had other random urine screens that were all negative, and since the additional one she requested was also negative, the Director could document the consistent absence of drugs and clear her. Interestingly, this same nurse was able to help investigate the diversion problem. Another nurse was identified and sent to treatment. Human nature being what it is, people who are known to have had problems will probably be the first ones suspected. But through monitoring we can provide firm documentation to dispel unjust accusations and can also discover a relapse.

Most programs around the country use several methods of monitoring simultaneously: 1) random urine or blood screens; 2) written reports from counselors/sponsors/employers; 3) self-reports written by the professional in recovery; and 4) written verification of attendance at mutual-help or support-group meetings. Each program may have its own unique design for governing how often monitoring is done, who does it, who follows up on identified problems, and the consequences and procedures in cases of noncompliance. Many state-level programs function under heavy budgetary restrictions and may not have adequate personnel to carry out much of the monitoring themselves. So they may delegate it to a combination of professional sponsors in the professional's geographic area, other treatment counselors providing aftercare, and the professional's employer. Regardless of who actually carries out the monitoring, it's usually processed by the state-level impairment or peer assistance program.

Body Fluid Monitoring

This country has developed a preoccupation with the legal and ethical ramifications of urine testing. For months it was impossible to pass a newsstand without seeing a cover story on drug testing. In recent years political candidates have volunteered for urine tests and challenged opponents to do the same. Issues of concern about urine testing in industry include several factors: 1) the violation of the individual's rights to privacy in testing body fluids, the methods of collection of the sample, and disclosure of the results of the testing; 2) determination of conditions that give the employer the right to request a urine sample; 3) chain-of-evidence procedures after the collection of the sample; and 4) determination of employers' rights to take action based on the results of the drug screen.

In monitoring the professional in recovery we too are concerned with the need for privacy and with careful chain-of-evidence procedures, but the decision that specimens will be obtained has been made, and intervals are already predetermined as random. The consequences of testing positive are defined in the agreement between the program and the professional. So this type of monitoring is quite different in that the person has already consented to the conditions of random testing in the program agreement or in the return-to-work contract. This monitoring isn't a fishing expedition designed to do initial case finding. The agreement also allows the monitor/employer to request a random urine screen when there's any question as to the stability of the professional in recovery, despite the fact that a screen may have been done only several days ago. In cases where the professional may have used drugs after the last random urine screen, the person may attempt to postpone the next collection for several days to give the drug time to be completely excreted in the urine. In this situation, the collector must be supportive but firm about the need for the specimen—**today.**

Whether the monitoring is done on blood or urine samples will depend on the basic program philosophy, primary drug abused, and whether tampering with the specimens is suspected. (See Appendix F.) Use of blood samples is certainly an invasive procedure and somewhat uncomfortable, and this may be a consideration in determining which method to use. Additionally, many persons in recovery (if they've been using intravenously) have few or no veins from which to draw the specimens, and this does present a problem. On the other hand, if one is an alcoholic in recovery and is suspected of having "slipped," the probability is that you won't find significant positive results in the urine but may well find measurable alcohol in the bloodstream. Blood may be preferred if it seems impossible to expect a carefully observed urine specimen. Social rather than physical reasons may make a collection totally impractical. In the long run, the usual method of monitoring is to use random observed urine samples. For those who are recovering from dependence on alcohol, both methods may be used, or a rotation of blood/urine samples may be used. If a relapse is suspected, it's advisable to test both blood and urine because blood testing gives more precise information about levels of the drug and how recently it was used.

Random Samples

When we say random, that's exactly what we mean. Whoever is doing the collecting should keep a chart or calendar listing with nonsequential dates on which to test the professionals, but that doesn't mean every other Tuesday/ Thursday or twice a month on Fridays at 3 p.m. The key to using drug screening wisely as a monitoring tool is its unpredictability. Schedule some requests for mornings, some for afternoons, some for before a day off, after a day off, or on a Saturday very soon after a previous collection. Through a truly random method you establish the credibility of the specimen. Some programs and employers require that several samples be collected each month, only some of which are sent for processing. For example, four specimens may be collected each month, but only one or two are sent for actual screening. This also increases the randomness of the testing and reduces the overall testing costs, and the professional can't anticipate which samples will actually be tested.

A recovering pharmacist who was being monitored by the local office of a disciplinary board told us that on the last Friday of every month he received a call to come down and give a urine specimen. This pattern was so predictable he could plan his life around it and of course could use drugs if he decided to. We recommend that you develop an individualized yearly graph for each professional you're monitoring and predetermine the dates for the random testing. This not only serves the obvious purpose but also reminds you to make a note on your calendar to remind you about obtaining the specimen.

Who Collects the Specimen?

There are numerous possibilities for deciding who will be the collector. Sometimes this task is delegated to a staff member at the treatment center, sometimes to a local professional in recovery who serves as a resource to the state program, sometimes to the employer, but always to one of the same sex as the recovering professional. Regardless of who that person is, the role shouldn't be switched back and forth among various people. It's embarrassing at best to give an observed specimen; providing the same collector makes the process a bit easier.

Ideally, the person who assumes this task won't have supervisory responsibility for the professional's practice nor the role of sponsor. Professionals often initially view the random urine screens as a process based on suspicion and as a reminder that they're not trusted, and these perceptions may work against the developing relationship between them and sponsors or therapists. In the work setting this responsibility may be naturally assumed by the employee health services without much difficulty. For confidentiality purposes, the person assigned to collecting the specimens may be told (with the professional's permission) that the person is in recovery and that drug screening is a standard part of the recovery. The only records that should be maintained by the collector are those of the actual laboratory reports and chain-of-evidence documentation; collectors don't need to know any of the details. Specimens are to be identified by code numbers only. Copies of the screening results should be provided to the professional in recovery and, if required, to a state-level program. The program gets a release form that gives the monitor permission to disclose results of the testing at the time of the professional's return to work and/or enrollment in a peer assistance or regulatory program.

Confidentiality

Many programs use a coding system to protect the professional's identity. This system must be in writing, and a key must be available to determine the name of the person assigned to that code number. This method ensures privacy as the specimen is received in the laboratory and results are reported. Legally it's not advisable to use fictitious names because there's no method to establish that the specimen belongs to the professional in recovery.

An incident was relayed to us about this very problem. A routine random urine sample was obtained from a physician in recovery, and the collector used a fictitious name on the laboratory slip to protect the physician's name. After twenty-four hours a report was phoned from the outside laboratory stating that both cocaine and opiates were present in the urine. This initial report created quite a crisis, and confirmation was requested by other laboratory testing methods. In the meantime, the monitor who had received the results called the doctor supervising the lab, requested that a second sample be tested, and notified the state program. Quite a few people were now involved. When the confirmation was called back, the monitor, still disbelieving the report, questioned the laboratory technician about the numbers on the lab slip to make sure they matched the log sheet in his office. At this point the mistake was discovered: The specimen belonged to another person with the same name as the common fictitious one invented for the physician. Granted, these situations are rare, but considering what's at stake it's best to use maximum safeguards.

Observed Collecting

Collecting an **observed** urine sample is the key to initiating the necessary chain-of-custody in urine testing. Chain-of-custody begins with actually witnessing the collection and handling the sample from the time it's provided by the professional in recovery and then sealed with a tamper-proof tape and placed in a tamper-resistant bag till the testing process is completed. Each person who handles the sample must document on the chain-of-custody form the time of the handling and disposition of the specimen. Unfortunately, many programs that monitor professionals in recovery don't use these often-cumbersome methods of handling; they simply label the specimen and send it to the laboratory. However, we live in a litigious society, so we must take appropriate measures to protect ourselves and the professional from any loss or substitution of specimens. It's becoming clearer that more programs will have to adopt these strict methods of collecting and transporting the specimens.

Some professionals have difficulty with the fact that direct observation is the recommended method for ensuring that the urine has not been altered, tampered with, substituted, or diluted. It may sound exaggerated, but those professionals who decide to beat the system are quite clever in preventing their drug use from being discovered. We're not saying that no people in early recovery can be trusted; we're saying that none of us should trust the disease itself. To be off guard helps no one. Checking the professional for presence of personal belongings, packages, and purses, and having these items at a distance when the specimen is given, observing the collection, and sealing and removing the sample from the professional immediately—all these measures help you deter several possible methods of altering the specimen:

1. Substituting someone else's urine sample contained in purse, knapsack, bag or vagina
2. Substituting urine from a hospitalized patient (urine brought to the collection area in a small bag)
3. Diluting the sample by adding water from the toilet bowl

Despite your observation the specimen may still have been provided by someone else. For example, when a male nurse was called to give a specimen he prepared a small bag of a patient's urine and attached small intravenous tubing to the plastic urine bag, which he secured under his arm. The tubing extended down his arm under his long-sleeved shirt, and when he went to give the specimen, he slipped the clamp open under his shirt and appearing to be urinating from the "right place," since his hand held the tip of the tubing and his penis at the same time!

When persons are at risk of exposure they do become ingenious, even desperate. One oft-repeated story tells of a physician who sat in his car outside the collecting site, catheterized his own bladder, removed his own urine, instilled his son's urine, then went in and gave his specimen under close observation. This was discovered only much later when he told the story himself.

Through effective procedures for collecting observed urines we identify problems early, rather than months down the road. Many experts advise that at the time the specimen is received from the subject it should be examined for color, temperature, and acidity to identify any gross abnormality. Normal urine has a yellow coloring; if it's very pale or almost colorless, this could indicate dilution. A fresh specimen of urine is warm from the body temperature; if it's cool, it may be a substituted specimen. One New York addict described giving urine where no one wished to demean anyone by invading privacy as it was collected. Men went one at a time into a bathroom where in plain sight on the radiator stood a large bottle labeled "Clean Urine. Help Yourself."

Acidity (or PH) of urine can be simply tested at the time of collection by dipping a special paper strip into the urine that will indicate by color change the acidity of the sample and also indicate if the sample may have been diluted or otherwise tampered with. Laboratories also should examine for gross physical properties, but they might not relay their suspicion that the sample was altered.

After being collected, the specimen should be secured with tape and initialed by the collector, and appropriate chain-of-custody and laboratory forms should be completed and enclosed with the specimen in a tamper-proof chain-of-custody transport bag. The professional in recovery should be asked if he or she is taking any prescribed medications or over-the-counter preparations; this information is recorded on the lab slip. Some programs require that persons in recovery initial a log sheet that indicates that it's their specimen that they observed being sealed and prepared.

Detecting the Presence of Alcohol

The use of urine screens for identifying the presence of alcohol isn't recommended, because little alcohol is excreted in the urine, and it's difficult to measure under normal circumstances. Monitoring for the presence of alcohol is most effectively done by obtaining a Blood Alcohol Concentration (B.A.C.). This procedure should also be performed according to strict protocol and chain-of-custody. Persons who don't frequently draw a B.A.C. may not be aware that the procedure calls for skin preparation at the injection site with other than the usual alcohol pads so as not to contaminate the specimen. Again, this test may reflect large amounts of over-the-counter preparations that contain alcohol, but people being monitored for alcohol aren't supposed to be taking anything containing alcohol. Many cough and cold preparations containing mind-altering drugs such as alcohol, antihistamines, or ephedrine are sold over the counter in grocery stores, drug stores, and convenience stores. Take a few minutes in your local drug store to read some ingredient labels, and see how difficult it is to select an item that has no potentially mind-altering drugs. One of us remembers the frustration of a nurse in recovery who had the flu and developed very bad chest congestion with uncontrollable fits of coughing. She went to the drugstore to get some cough medicine, only to find that almost all the available preparations in that store contained alcohol or another forbidden drug. She did finally find a product with the help of the pharmacist, but it wasn't easy.

Dealing with Positive Laboratory Results

(Refer to Appendix F for types of testing.)
When the final laboratory report confirms a positive result on a recovering professional:

1. If the confirmation method wasn't by GC/MS (again, see Appendix F), request that this test be run on the original urine specimen (most laboratories hold specimens for about a month).
2. Request a second specimen from the professional and again ask if he or she is taking any over-the-counter medications. Be meticulous in collecting, and observe completely. Use proper chain-of-custody procedures, coding to ensure confidentiality, and divide the specimen into two containers.
3. Send one sample to the original laboratory for retesting, using the same procedures for screening and confirmation.
4. Send the second sample to a different laboratory for similar testing.

The important thing to remember about drug screening is that it's merely a tool, not a diagnostic measure of recovery (or of relapse). If you receive positive results, don't panic; simply follow the procedures outlined and await confirmation before jumping into action. When you receive final results and still have questions, you may wish to contact the laboratory's medical director or consultant and have that person review the case with you and discuss the reliability of the tests used.

A dentist in recovery was required to submit random urine samples to the state board to document her recovery during a two-year probationary period. For a year and a half she had never had a positive urine, and her recovery was confirmed by reports from the treatment professionals providing her after-care. During her last six months of probation, the monitor ran the usual random urine screen. It came back positive for marijuana. The test was repeated on the first specimen, and a second urine sample was sent for testing. The second results were even higher than the first! A sample of the specimen was then sent (by special request) to an out-of-state laboratory that specialized in drug screening, and it was tested by GC/MS with a negative result. After much investigation and consultation, it was discovered that, at the time of the urine screening, the nurse was taking large amounts of ibuprofen for a painful shoulder injury and that this had yielded a false positive in the testing. Apparently, in large quantities the ibuprofen (Advil, Nuprin, Medipren) may mimic marijuana by-products like THC and show as a positive reading on chromatography.

When selecting your laboratory you may request listings of substances that may alter drug screening so that you're prepared to think logically and calmly if you receive positive results on a professional in recovery. Just remember that the same list is available to the subject. That's why one should ask at the time of the collection about medications, if any, that have been recently used.

Here are the guidelines for random urine screening.
1. Develop a schedule for "random testing."
2. Each month send 50% of the collected urines for actual screening.
3. A professional of the same sex directly observes the collection of each sample.
4. The collector examines the urine for color, temperature, and acidity.
5. Record on the lab slip any over-the-counter preparations or current prescription medication.
6. Follow the chain-of-custody procedure.
7. Ensure confidentiality by coding on laboratory slips.
8. A designated professional receives the reports.
9. Provide copies of reports to the professional in recovery and to the program if required.
10. Maintain records of urine screening in a locked file accessible only to the monitor.

Monitoring Through Reports

Most programs for impaired professionals have some form of monitoring that includes written reports as primary documentation of continuing progress and recovery. If the program was notified and involved at the time of intervention, the professional may already have received paperwork from the program while in treatment and may have completed the necessary agreements and release forms before discharge. If so, the program may request a copy of the discharge plan and communicate with the aftercare counselor to explain the program's procedure for submitting progress reports. Each program may differ in the frequency of the reporting and the title of the person reporting, but someone other than the professional in recovery is documenting the professional's current status and progress for the program. The program may have its own required report forms that it sends to specified persons. Some programs' philosophy may be that it's the responsibility of the professional in recovery to ensure that the counselors or employers send in the evaluations at the proper time.

Most programs have defined guidelines for the written monitoring procedures and adhere to their policies. Many programs regard tardiness in sending reports as lack of responsibility on the part of the professional in recovery and send written notifications that the required documentation hasn't been received by the agreed date. When it's been determined that the professional isn't following through on the required reporting, the program may notify the person that continued delinquency in submitting the documentation may result in termination from the program. Sometimes the professional in recovery is put in the position of having to force an employer who procrastinates to send reports to the program. It's never easy for such a person to get a superior to act, and if this is the situation the professional should discuss it with someone (such as the program director or coordinator) who can help early on so that the professional won't be in the position of offering explanations long after the papers are due. It's also common for professionals in recovery to lose sight of the primary function of the program (to ensure safety of practice while providing advocacy to the professional) and to express resentment about the program's insistence on monitoring their recovery. These persons newly in recovery do need structure and specified limits, both of which are provided by discharge planning and program agreements; but predictably their enthusiasm about compliance may wax and wane.

Programs for impaired professionals may request reports from other professionals (such as the following) who have consistent contact with the person in recovery:

1. Counselor: the primary aftercare counselor who sees the person regularly in groups and/or individually during recovery. This aftercare counselor may also be responsible for initiating the random urine screens.
2. Monitor: usually another professional in recovery but with longtime sobriety who agrees to provide support and monitoring to the person newly in recovery. Many physician programs use local monitors who can provide leadership in recovery and can document the professional's progress.
3. Employer: Many programs require either monthly or quarterly reports from the professional's employer. Ideally, one person accepts this ongoing responsibility. Providing consistency in evaluating progress and performance means less subjectivity in reporting progress and

greater opportunity for developing a trusting relationship between the professional in recovery and the employer.

4. Self-reports: Many state programs require professionals in recovery to submit monthly self-reports describing their status, their progress, and in general how they're feeling about themselves. Having had the opportunity to review hundreds of such letters, we believe that these are the most revealing of all required reports. For persons who have great difficulty expressing their feelings, this is a valuable therapeutic experience. The letters often express deep feelings, fears, concerns, and insights and when read carefully may give a very accurate picture of recovery. Many program participants develop an emotional relationship with the program through the required self-reports. There is relatively little fear of rejection, since "They already know my worst secret." This attitude enhances subjects' willingness to be self-disclosing in their letters.

For some, this monthly task becomes an opportunity to share thoughts and feelings about themselves and about the recovery process that they otherwise might not be able to identify till months later. When these letters indicate preoccupation with the drug of choice, frequent dreams about the drug, inability to cope, depression, or even desire to give up the professional licensure, they may be regarded as signals warning that the person could relapse. Check to see if the counselors, the employer, colleagues, or the sponsor have picked up signs of impending relapse or serious depression. If so, resources can be quickly mobilized to provide the professional with reassurance and intensive counseling to help him or her through this difficult period. In some programs when the professional in recovery appears at risk for relapse, a program employee may call promptly to offer reassurance and support and get a firsthand, personal view of the situation.

Medical Illness in Recovery

Professionals in recovery aren't immune to the illnesses or conditions experienced by others in recovery. They may need extensive dental or surgical treatment. They suffer injuries and illnesses requiring pain medications or other mind-altering drugs. It's common to hear healthcare professionals express the belief that "addicts shouldn't have any prescription pain medication," and medical and nursing staff may foolishly attempt to alleviate severe pain with inadequate nonprescription pain relievers. Professionals with special needs should be placed under the care of physicians who understand chemical dependence and who can administer narcotics and other potentially addictive drugs when appropriate.

General Healthcare Recommendations

Professionals in recovery should investigate resources within their communities for receiving dental and medical care from professionals knowledgeable about chemical dependence. Some may themselves be in recovery. It's important that we realize the risk of relapse after a professional in recovery receives drugs or anesthesia and that we take appropriate measures to reduce this risk. When it's not feasible to have a healthcare provider who's well-informed about chemical dependence, it's still strongly recommended that persons in recovery put their physicians and dentists in touch with another medical professional within the community who's knowledgeable about chemical dependence and who can serve as a consultant and resource during their treatment. This is a must! Most healthcare providers have limited knowledge of chemical dependence and don't know how to provide effective pain relief while also protecting their patients against relapse. In some communities, physicians who are medical directors of chemical dependence treatment centers serve as consultants to other physicians, as do some physicians who are advocates for the state-level impairment programs. Every professional in recovery should seek out these resource people.

Outpatient Procedures

The most common outpatient treatment that may require pain relief is dental work. As more sophisticated procedures are performed in the office, the patient may need moderate pain medication for the first twelve to twenty-four hours. If a patient newly in recovery requires a drug or anesthesia, it's advisable that the person be accompanied to the office by a colleague or sponsor in recovery who will offer support and reassurance while it's wearing off. Ideally, these support people will take the professional home and stay there (if the person lives alone) for the first twenty-four hours after the person has been given the drug or anesthesia.

If even oral pain medication is needed, it's advisable to consult with the identified medical consultant about which medication to use and the recommended dose. The prescription should always be limited to the number of pills normally required for severe pain relief during the first few days. Instructions should also be given to the colleague, friend, or sponsor who's with the person that someone other than the professional (for instance, a colleague or family member) should if possible be responsible for dispensing the pills. Persons in recovery who are taking pain medication or who have just undergone medical procedures should increase their meeting attendance and aftercare counseling and be encouraged to talk about the feelings they had while taking the drug. The goal is to take as little of the pain medication as possible, to look carefully at any unusual amounts or prolonged use of the medication, and to be aware that such drugs can alter judgment and perception.

Hospitalized Patients in Recovery

Many persons in recovery feel great anxiety about undergoing surgery. They fear that if they disclose they're in recovery the staff may withhold adequate amounts of pain medication. Considering the attitudes and ignorance that exist, their fears are well founded. However, by obtaining a physician who has expertise in chemical dependence or is willing to work with a chemical dependence consultant, their fears can be alleviated. Depending upon which drugs they used heavily while active in their addiction, recommendations will be made regarding which type of pain relief might be most effective and what dose would be required for relief.

It's also recommended that while they're hospitalized they have sponsors and colleagues in recovery present even outside normal visiting hours to offer support while they're receiving the medications or to help them through the transition from injections to oral medication and through the gradual change to nonnarcotic pain relievers. Keep in mind that by administering the drugs we may be activating the disease of chemical dependence and that the person may be tempted to request medication when it's not really necessary, or may attempt to get someone to increase the medication without accurately assessing the relief received from the current dose. Again, this is an area where the colleague in recovery can render invaluable assistance in helping the person to assess his or her need for the medication and in offering some diversion from any preoccupation that might be developing.

The key to treating the professional in recovery who has been administered anesthesia or other drugs during hospitalization is to allow the person to detoxify from them while still in the hospital. Ideally, such persons shouldn't be discharged until twenty-four hours after any narcotics (even mild ones taken orally) are discontinued. In an age of stringent insurance reimbursement, this is becoming an increasingly difficult task but should be strongly considered.

Relapse

Chemical dependence is a chronic, primary, progressive disease that is treatable. Left untreated, it's usually fatal. Like other chronic illnesses it's subject to relapse, even after treatment. The disease can be tenacious despite aggressive efforts at treatment and sincere efforts at recovery. Relapse does happen, but it's not a reason to give up! Many professionals who have intervened with colleagues mistakenly feel personal failure in the event of relapse, get angry, or lose faith in intervention and treatment if there's not total success after the first attempt.

It's easy to write off the impaired person and walk away feeling disappointed, resentful, and frustrated. Would it be as easy to turn away from a diabetic who had been under good control and suddenly developed symptoms of acidosis? Clearly, the difference lies in our understanding and acceptance of the disease and our experiences with it through our clinical practice. We know that diabetes is managed with insulin and diet, but we do expect that at times control will be lost again and that more aggressive treatment will be needed. Through experience healthcare providers **accept** their inability to "cure" the diabetes and learn to focus their energies on providing the person with therapy that may lengthen his or her time in control and increase life expectancy.

Unfortunately, many professional people lack similar experience with chemical dependence and haven't had the opportunity of accepting its chronic and progressive course. Without this acceptance it's very difficult, if not impossible, to give the best part of themselves to their recovering colleagues who desperately need encouragement. Actually, the outlook isn't at all gloomy. Generally, professionals who receive treatment have a better-than-average chance of staying sober. Even those who relapse once after treatment and get right back into a recovery program do well. Three major factors account for that: They usually fear the loss of licensure, they get involved in follow-up treatment, and they benefit from careful monitoring. In short, we should be neither pessimistic nor complacent about their recovery. What's important is to be alert for possible relapse, have a plan for handling it, and go into action promptly if it happens or if we suspect it.

Relapse is generally thought of as going back to using alcohol/other drugs. But certain subtle changes can occur before a person actually starts using drugs again. As a matter of fact, people in recovery do seem to relapse **without** using drugs. A typical dictionary definition of the verb "relapse" is "to slip back into a former state." The "former state" for professionals in recovery certainly involved many complicated emotional dynamics aside from the alcohol/other drug use. These persons often revert to old patterns of distorted perceptions and old defense mechanisms. They get uncomfortable and attempt to avoid dealing with personal or professional issues that are unpleasant or anxiety-producing. Remember, these persons relied heavily on drugs to make them feel better, and they avoided unpleasant situations by using drugs. These changes generally develop gradually, but the more people try to dissociate from the relationships and life issues at hand, the more complicated those things become, until eventually not dealing with things snowballs and they can't handle the situation. It's common to see professionals in this type of emotional relapse exhibit other compulsive behaviors such as spending or buying impulsively, overeating, or gambling. During an **emotional relapse** some exhibit behavioral changes and show unpredictable mood swings, are depressed or irritable, withdraw from co-workers, and express resentment toward the demands of recovery, including monitoring and counseling. This relapse may then extend to gradual missing of aftercare meetings (with elaborate excuses), hopping from one A.A. group to another despite developed relationships with their "home group," designing their own recovery program (deciding what **they'll** do and when), resisting sending monthly reports to the designated program and/or gradually sending them later and later, and avoiding recovering colleagues and sponsors. A.A. members often call this a "dry drunk."

When the behaviors of emotional relapse have been identified, more intervention is appropriate and may be initiated by a professional such as yourself, a concerned employer, primary counselor, or another colleague in recovery. These interventions need not be elaborate and are highly successful in reestablishing reality for the professional. What we need to do is to point out, again through objective data, that all is not well, make sure the treatment and support people already involved are fully aware of the situation, and insist that the person follow both existing treatment plans and new suggestions, should new ones be necessary.

A **relapse with alcohol/other drugs** predictably may follow an emotional relapse—particularly, of course, if the emotional relapse is ignored. In rare instances it may occur suddenly, seemingly with no warning. Relapse can be identified in a variety of ways, but in many cases it's reported spontaneously by the professional, particularly by one involved in a formal program. Those who don't report can be identified by colleagues, who usually can observe changes in behavior. These people are experiencing a heavy sense of guilt and failure, so we needn't add to the burden by blaming them or reproaching them no matter how tempting it is to start with "After all I've done for you . . ."

Those who self-report are often in a state of severe anxiety and need reassurance and direction. They may report to you immediately after the alcohol/other drug use that places them at high risk for impulsive reaction. At all costs, avoid any expression of judgment, rejection, or disappointment. Those dealing with the relapse must provide support, understanding, and acceptance, but don't ignore it or keep it secret. No relapse is trivial.

A nurse who was six months in recovery had been undergoing some questionable "personality changes" that were reported by her supervisors and colleagues to the state-level program. After receiving similar reports from the primary treatment counselor, the state program director suggested that an intervention take place with the primary counselor, employer, and a colleague in recovery. The day before the planned intervention, the nurse injected 400 mg of Demerol intravenously while at work but called the state program immediately afterward. She told what she had done and asked for help. While one employee kept her on the phone and offered support and reassurance, another called her employer and directed the employer to go to the floor from which the nurse was calling. The employer arrived, and a three-way conversation was held to explain what had happened. The employer was willing to help and did so. Arrangements were made for the nurse to be escorted at once to an inpatient facility for evaluation of this episode and for subsequent treatment.

When a professional relapses, he or she should immediately be relieved of professional responsibilities and evaluated by the primary counselor and the treatment team. Some who relapse may not be able to stop on their own, so it's advisable to admit them for evaluation while assuring them a supportive, safe environment. For those who relapse by taking even one drink or one of someone else's tranquilizers or medications, immediate evaluation is critical. If they have adequate supports and resources in their home and community, and if the alcohol/other drug use didn't continue, outpatient evaluation should usually suffice. Depending on the circumstances of the relapse, the treatment team may make a variety of recommendations, including increasing attendance at aftercare and 12-Step meetings, individual counseling sessions, changes in professional responsibility or work environment, or additional inpatient treatment. When the final recommendations are made it may be necessary to hold a formal meeting with the treatment team, the professional, the employer, and/or the program representative to reinforce the need for compliance with the treatment recommendations and to offer support and encouragement to the professional. At this point a new contract may be initiated that outlines the updated treatment plan, employment expectations and limitations, and program stipulations. The relapsed professional is often extremely depressed and devoid of any energy to argue with the recommendations. The same safety precautions outlined in Chapter 6 (under The Risk of Suicide) should be taken when dealing with the relapse.

The key to addressing relapse effectively is to **act**, not to wait until you're **sure** something is wrong. The simple fact that you suspect something is amiss demonstrates the need to:

1. Assess the professional's behaviors and begin data collection
2. Coordinate intervention with primary counselors/treatment professionals
3. Do a timely intervention

In our experience, relapse is quite manageable if you're not astonished or caught off guard. Avoid extremes. Don't overreact and take impulsive, ill-conceived action. But don't minimize what has happened. Take any relapse seriously. If you ignore it, you signal at once that a little bit of drinking or taking another drug now and then is really all right—and you pave the way to disaster. Remember: In spite of the relapse, you're well ahead of where you were before the intervention, and you'll be doing similar, familiar things.

Life Begins with Intervention

The following are selected case examples of chemically dependent professionals who were identified and successfully intervened with by colleagues. In committing these stories to print we're reminded not only of the powerful feelings of sadness and disbelief felt by colleagues of the impaired professionals before intervention, but also of the sense of celebration that surrounds their entry into recovery.

Case 1

Mary was a registered nurse with many years' clinical experience in large teaching hospitals. She was married and had three children; her husband John was a sales manager for a hospital supply company and frequently traveled. Mary worked during the daytime hours and arranged for childcare for her children after school until she could pick them up.

Mary was employed at the same hospital for five years and was well liked by colleagues, who described her as "quiet and very sweet to the patients." During her employment her performance appraisals were always above average, and she was twice offered the position of charge nurse, which she refused, saying, "I really don't want to leave bedside nursing." Her friends at work admired her not only for her nursing expertise but also for her ability to manage both a full-time career and a family.

During the spring of her fifth year of employment, several incidents raised some concerns among colleagues. She began arriving late to work, which was very unusual for her, and had various reasons for her tardiness. When she did arrive, she appeared disorganized and had a difficult time setting priorities for her patient care. Over several months Mary began calling in sick or claiming the kids were sick. These sick days began to show a pattern that coincided with her days off.

Mary's care of her patients was also undergoing subtle changes. She was increasingly forgetting to change medication orders, and several of her charts contained inappropriate nursing notes. She also was pulling away from any contact with her friends and co-workers.

When the head nurse received several patient complaints about Mary, she began collecting information from her colleagues and requested their observations in written form.

Mary arrived at work twenty minutes late one morning, looking pale and shaky. The head nurse detected the odor of alcohol on her breath, questioned her about it, and asked Mary to go to the Employee Health Service to be checked by the physician before working. Mary readily agreed and went as requested. Meanwhile, the head nurse notified the Employee Health Service of her suspicion about Mary's alcohol use and requested that they delay seeing her until the head nurse could contact the peer assistance program.

Peer assistance sent a liaison to the hospital to meet with the head nurse and the supervisor. When the information had been reviewed it was recommended that an intervention take place in the Employee Health Services after an examination by the physician and a voluntary blood alcohol-level test. Mary agreed to the blood sample and was examined while the intervention team was preparing to intervene. Included in the intervention were her head nurse, nursing administrator, a friend from work, a nurse in recovery, and the peer assistance liaison. After Mary's examination she was brought to an office in the Employee Health Services where the intervention team was gathered. The intervention followed the format outlined in this book, although Mary didn't argue or challenge. She admitted to "drinking too much lately" (her blood alcohol test was positive) and wanted help. Of course, this isn't the usual response, but Mary was experiencing the painful physical effects of the alcohol as well as the tremendous leverage presented by the team—her employment and potentially her license. She agreed to go to inpatient evaluation and treatment (if recommended).

Mary completed a 28-day treatment program with flying colors. At the time of her intervention, she was clearly in a crucial phase of chemical dependence that was beginning to destroy her personal and professional life.

Her husband, who also was suspected by the treatment team of being alcoholic, refused to participate in the family program. With the support of the treatment team and intensive individual counseling, Mary separated from her actively alcoholic husband and resumed employment at the same hospital on a different nursing unit.

Two years later, Mary serves as a contact person for the peer assistance program and helps support groups for chemically dependent nurses.

Case 2

Lily was a thirty-nine-year-old pediatrician who worked as a full-time salaried hospital employee. She had given up her office and private practice some years ago when demands of husband and children forced her to take a position with more predictable hours. She had no second job. She and her husband had separated three years earlier, and her adolescent son, Teddy, still lived at home with her; her other two children were off at college. Lily seemed to manage the breakup of her marriage without undue distress and until recently had been accepted and admired as a competent woman who enjoyed her life and met its inevitable challenges with humor and flexibility.

But then Lily began to seem preoccupied. She looked tired and strained and was short with friends who asked if everything was all right. She dropped out of a regular weekly bridge group and vanished from the circle of fellow pediatricians with whom she had regularly shared a cocktail and shop talk. There were rumors that Teddy was having trouble in school and that Lily was having financial problems attributed to college expenses for the two older children and a husband who was cavalier at best about support payments.

Lily's work performance remained adequate but rather minimal. She did what she was hired to do but very little more, left for home as soon as her work was finished, and stopped staying late to teach the medical students and house staff, something she had much enjoyed and that had made her a great favorite.

Nursing staff discovered that narcotics were missing, compared notes with one another, and started watching very carefully for any unauthorized people who might have contact with opiates. Lily twice volunteered to give injections for a nurse who was busy when an older child was allegedly impatient for pain relief. However, the child said he had not asked for or received a shot on either occasion. Finally, Lily was seen taking a filled syringe that briefly had been left unattended.

At a hastily arranged intervention, Lily adamantly refused to admit to using drugs. Only when threatened with a report to a disciplinary board and termination from the hospital on the spot did she agree to go to evaluation. After admission, she volunteered almost nothing and continued to deny any problem. She gave in only when it was made clear that unless she could be candid, the report of the theft that had been observed and couldn't be explained away was indeed going to be reported.

It developed that she didn't use and never had used drugs. Her son Teddy had developed a serious and expensive narcotic addiction, and he had persuaded her to keep this secret so as not to jeopardize his reputation and chances of getting into college. They had agreed that she would bring home opiates from work and would taper him off and detoxify him at home. Then he would go into treatment with a good psychotherapist. But some months later Teddy was still using opiates at much the same level as before. Lily couldn't tell anyone the story without also admitting her own foolishness and her diversion of drugs.

She required a great deal of reeducation before she was able to stop enabling her son and to get him into treatment. Fortunately she didn't lose her license.

Her situation taught us yet again that not everything that looks at first glance like an obvious addiction is just that. We know that chemical dependence in the family can affect every one of its members, but it's rarely so easy to demonstrate.

Case 3

Robert was a trial lawyer, a senior member of his firm, well respected for his brilliance and inventiveness. He was popular and active in his community, and friends had often tried to persuade him to run for public office—suggestions that pleased him but that he dismissed, since he enjoyed his present work and valued his time with his children.

Every year seemed to bring new successes until, when he was in his late thirties, his drinking became increasingly frequent, began earlier in the day, and later continued during work hours. He kept a bottle in his desk drawer and began to take an extra nip before going to court or meeting with a new client.

His colleagues responded by manipulating his schedule so that work requiring maximum alertness appeared on his morning schedule and less and less was expected of him in the afternoons. Even with his increasing limitations, he seemed always able to rise to the occasion, and when he was working well he remained so productive that he easily caught up with whatever he had postponed.

He became involved in the case of a friend, a businessman charged with second-degree murder supposedly committed while he was drinking heavily during Mardi Gras. Robert took the case and agreed to go to New Orleans to locate and interview an alibi witness. Instead, he began to drink as soon as he arrived there and ultimately went on a prolonged binge that consumed the time and money available for his task. After making half-hearted and unsuccessful efforts to locate the witness, he returned home to New England, convinced that by charm, skill, and persuasiveness he could win the case without the witness. The trial took place, and his friend was convicted and jailed.

Robert drank.

Finally, nearly a year later, after a DWI arrest and a front-page report of a drunken brawl in which Robert was involved, his colleagues called for help from members of a Lawyers Concerned for Lawyers group. Several of them appeared, did an effective intervention, and maneuvered Robert into residential treatment. He was able to get sober and is still actively involved in A.A.

Recovery as a Journey

Recovery is a lifelong process for the chemically dependent professional. This chronic disease requires a continuing investment in staying well. The journey of recovery is one of gaining personal insight and spiritual strength and of fellowship with others in recovery, and the process is never completed. There's no day when one is "all fixed up"; recovery is a path of unfolding self-knowledge, awareness, and sensitivity that helps a person to experience life fully.

Treatment, in the broad sense, usually should last for about two years, with more treatment as necessary, sometimes continuing without interruption, sometimes at intervals as new problems arise. Mutual support groups like A.A. and N.A. shouldn't be regarded as a form of treatment to be completed but as the fellowship they really are, available for a lifetime.

There will never be a "cure" in the sense that an alcoholic can ever return safely to social drinking or another drug addict can return to an injection now and then. But these people can live fully and comfortably without alcohol/other drugs in a world full of them and of people who use them.

Long after program participation has ended or aftercare is completed, the professional continues in recovery and keeps the relationships established during the initial recovery plan.

Recovery is **life** for these people. Through your compassion and reaching out to them when they're far from easy to love, you can give them the greatest gift of all.

Chapter Highlights

This final chapter has presented a variety of considerations regarding the treatment, aftercare, return to work, monitoring, and recovery of the chemically dependent professional. Some of the key points were:

Types of treatment available:
1. Inpatient: usually a minimum of 28 days in a facility specializing in chemical dependence treatment
2. Outpatient: formal chemical dependence treatment conducted daily/ weekly while the person remains in his or her normal life situation and perhaps continues employment
3. Extended treatment: inpatient chemical dependence treatment from three months to two years; may include gradual rehabilitation processes such as halfway houses and gainful employment
4. Aftercare: extension of the inpatient treatment process that continues on an outpatient basis for approximately one to two years at a formal chemical dependence treatment center

Discharge planning:
1. Coordinate with treatment team's recommendations.
2. Determine feasibility of return to practice.
3. Clarify limitations of practice imposed by state programs or by treatment recommendations.
4. Explore employment alternatives that are beneficial to both professional and employer.
5. Draft contracts to be presented before discharge.
6. Participate in discharge conference and offer support and reassurance.

Monitoring by random urine screens:
1. Develop a "random schedule" for testing.
2. Send 50% of samples per month (if more than one is collected) for actual screening.
3. Have same-sex monitor directly observe collection of sample.
4. Examine urine for color and temperature, and test for acidity.
5. Note any over-the-counter products the professional in recovery is currently taking.
6. Follow chain-of-custody procedures.
7. Ensure confidentiality.
8. Distribute reports of screening appropriately.

9. Provide the professional in recovery with copies of reports.
10. Maintain records of urine screening in a locked file accessible only to the monitor.

In the event of relapse:
1. Assess the behaviors and begin data collection.
2. Coordinate with primary counselor and treating professionals.
3. Do a timely intervention.

Medical illness during recovery:
1. Identify a medical professional with expertise in chemical dependence.
2. Seek medical professionals who are themselves in recovery (for example, dentists, physicians, anesthesiologists).
3. Provide colleague support during outpatient procedures.
4. Delegate dispensing of mind-altering medications to a family member or colleague.
5. Limit quantity of prescribed medications dispensed.
6. Provide sponsorship to professionals in recovery who are hospitalized.
7. Detoxify the professional before discharge.

Appendix A

Forms of Treatment

Chemical dependence treatment today typically takes four common forms: 1) inpatient treatment (generally lasting four weeks and usually including any necessary detoxification as part of a single admission); 2) extended or long-term residential treatment, usually lasting three months to a year; 3) outpatient treatment, usually for one to two years; and 4) "aftercare," a component usually designed to follow inpatient or outpatient treatment and lasting for one to two years. A full discussion of each of these types, their merits and disadvantages, would be well beyond the scope or purpose of this book. We'll attempt simply to present a brief description of each as it applies to treating impaired professionals. Many treatment providers in the field of chemical dependence hold opinions contrary to ours; however, our beliefs are held in common with many colleagues who have extensive expertise in intervention, evaluation, treatment, and monitoring of impaired professionals.

Inpatient Treatment

This is by far the most effective method of dealing with an impaired professional, particularly if the person is really being pushed into treatment under protest. Through denial and colleagues' enabling the impaired professional frequently reaches a late stage of the disease before intervention and therefore needs the structure and supportive environment of the inpatient setting. We've already mentioned the risk of suicide and the fact that families of these professionals often are enablers. For the patient, living in a home that's not ready to support recovery places him or her under considerable stress, and trying to comply with an outpatient treatment program and to manage alone in the face of a family's nonacceptance and even active subversion of the recovery process is an unnecessary handicap. Even with so much to lose, though, the professional will still often attempt to manipulate treatment, and it's usually easier to do this on an outpatient basis because neither the counseling staff nor the other patients can monitor much of what the patient does.

Clearly another advantage of the inpatient setting is that we've removed the professional from all other distractions, including the availability of alcohol/other drugs and the presence of those who use them. This gives him or her the freedom to focus on the primary tasks of understanding and accepting the disease of chemical dependence and working at recovery. In this safe, supportive environment the patient can more easily face and come to terms with the losses, changes, and other problems that are already there and those that lie ahead. Keep in mind that inpatient treatment is also desirable because some disciplinary bodies don't take kindly to chemical dependents in the first place, and they're less than supportive with those who fail to take full advantage of proffered treatment and go on to relapse. For some impaired professionals the first chance may be the only chance of staying in the profession, so one shouldn't start by cutting corners and making only minimal efforts, on the assumption that if such efforts fail, inpatient treatment can be tried next time. There may not be a next time.

In selecting an inpatient treatment center a number of criteria should be considered:

1. Does the medical director have demonstrated expertise in chemical dependence?
2. Are the counselors certified in treating chemical dependence?
3. Is there a balance of treatment staff that includes both those in recovery and others?
4. Does the center's philosophy include an introduction to Alcoholics Anonymous, Narcotics Anonymous, and other appropriate mutual self-help groups? Does the center refer clients to support groups specifically for professional people? (See Appendix H on resources.)
5. Is there a structured family program that the impaired professional's family can participate in?
6. Is aftercare provided or carefully arranged for at least one, ideally two, years?
7. Is the philosophy of recovery based on abstinence from all mind-altering drugs?
8. Can the center meet the needs of specific groups such as women, gays, ethnic minorities, and older adults?
9. Is the cost reasonable and covered by insurance?
10. Will any length of stay beyond four weeks really be determined by individual need and not at the whim of the treatment center staff?

Some well-established programs—Florida's, for example—have developed their own criteria for appropriate treatment of the impaired professional.

But without specific legislation and regulatory support such criteria could be challenged as arbitrary and prejudiced. Sometimes they are. If treatment choices are limited there probably won't be an optimal match between patient and facility. Having a list of approved treatment centers can eliminate places that sound very attractive on paper but that are much better at marketing than at treatment. Without formal guidelines, you and your impaired professional will be best served if you choose treatment centers on the basis of the criteria just listed.

Outpatient Treatment

Partially as a result of nationwide efforts to raise awareness of alcohol/other drug problems, there has been a huge increase in the demand for and establishment of treatment facilities. Many of them are outpatient clinics; some of them are day or evening programs in hospitals. Some are hospital-based; some are attached to freestanding residential treatment centers; others function totally independently. In an era of rapid change within the healthcare insurance industry, outpatient centers have attempted to meet the needs of chemically dependent persons who don't require inpatient treatment, who may not have coverage for inpatient treatment, or whose coverage is limited to only a very few days for detoxification but who do have benefits for outpatient counseling or psychiatric treatment.

Outpatient treatment is also an opportunity for employers who hope to provide recommended care at a significantly reduced cost. Sometimes very expensive care in hospitals is covered by insurance, but less expensive freestanding facilities and outpatient care isn't. For persons enrolled in outpatient treatment, there's less disruption of everyday life. They live at home and may continue to work or go to school while receiving treatment. Some of these outpatient arrangements by no means represent an easy commitment, since structured programs may require attendance up to six days per week and evenings in addition to regular attendance at mutual-support group meetings, but for some they're an acceptable and affordable alternative to inpatient treatment.

There are certain disadvantages to outpatient treatment. The intensive treatment phase may take longer than anticipated, and the person may get no relief from the stresses of everyday life (stresses that inpatient treatment can relieve by removing the patient from the everyday environment). Also, the person in outpatient treatment has much easier access to alcohol/other drugs. Acting impulsively, the person can easily drink or use again even while struggling to participate in the treatment program. In some circumstances and depending on which drugs the person has been using, disulfiram (Antabuse) and naltrexone (Trexan) can be used in conjunction with outpatient treatment to block the possibility of any satisfactory use of alcohol or opiates respectively and to enforce a "clean and dry" condition. This provides a very effective pharmacological straitjacket. However, those drugs are useless to those whose drug of choice is something other than alcohol or opiates, such as cocaine, marijuana, or tranquilizers.

Persons who are diagnosed in the early stages of the disease of chemical dependence or who are seeking help spontaneously can often do very well on an outpatient basis. However, we haven't arrived at the level of diagnostic sophistication required to reach people at the first signs of chemical dependence, and we may not do so for years. Meanwhile, it's almost impossible to force or to persuade into treatment many whom we can recognize very early. They can still say truthfully that they haven't been in any overt trouble with their careers, their outside relationships, violations for DWI or DUI, and suchlike. So it's safe to say that most professionals with whom we're forced to do interventions aren't likely to be candidates for outpatient programs, no matter how intensive those programs purport to be.

One of us remembers, early in her experience in this work, meeting a nurse who had twice lost her license for diverting Demerol and who was then working in a clerical job. She was still under the treatment of a psychiatrist and had twice been in psychiatric hospitals after having diverted narcotics and been fired. She hadn't used any drugs for nine months but obviously needed chemical dependence treatment. An outpatient program was recommended to her. She complied with its recommendations and successfully completed the program. Her license was reinstated at the urging of the treatment program and of other professionals working in the field of chemical dependence.

Soon after receiving her license again she exhibited troubling behavior: poor judgment, irritability, and outbursts of temper. She withdrew from colleagues and friends and began calling in sick to work. She was exhibiting some signs and symptoms of active chemical dependence, but she wasn't using Demerol and had no access to it where she worked. However, she **had** begun drinking. When confronted, she agreed to inpatient treatment, realizing that she now risked losing her license permanently. After completing six weeks in treatment she said, "If I'd done this in the first place, I wouldn't have lost my license the second time."

Of course, this may have been the wisdom of hindsight, but there was truth in what she was saying. Essentially, this last episode wasn't a relapse. Her disease of chemical dependence was activated again because it hadn't been fully addressed during two inpatient psychiatric admissions nor during the outpatient program. She admitted that she had remained in denial throughout the outpatient program and had merely complied with the treatment requirements in order to get her license back. Not until her inpatient treatment did she surrender to and accept that she was chemically dependent. It could certainly be argued that since she had started at the clinic without being in any crisis and with nine drug-free months behind her, her denial might have stayed intact no matter what the setting until some new event forced her to reevaluate her whole situation.

Long-Term (Extended) Residential Treatment

For a variety of reasons, some patients need more than 28-day programs can offer. The degree of brain damage (although most of this resolves with time) or the persistent lack of insight and of commitment to the hard work of maintaining abstinence may require a structured environment with ongoing therapy for anywhere from two months to two years. Some programs automatically recommend extended residential treatment for specific groups of professionals, particularly those in healthcare. These programs claim that treating chemical dependence requires intensive efforts well beyond the insurance-limited thirty days. Some of them use and sometimes maintain halfway houses as opportunities for the professional in recovery to interact and receive feedback from colleagues, to assume life responsibilities gradually, and perhaps to obtain a job, though not always in their field of expertise. Professionals learn to function effectively in this familylike environment while receiving limited ongoing therapy from counselors and support from colleagues in recovery.

Recommendation for this extended residential treatment will usually be made by the treatment team at the end of the four-week program. Sometimes it will be obvious much sooner that more time will be needed, and efforts may immediately be made to sell the patient on the idea. If you're wondering why the person is sent somewhere else rather than stay longer at the first center, the answer is usually because of lack of insurance. There are other reasons as well. Chemical dependence programs have well-defined sequential tracks that are the framework of the treatment. For example, the impaired professional will first complete Week One track of therapy, education, focus groups and such, before progressing to Weeks Two and Three. The program tracks conclude at Week Four. Most health-insurance policies have traditionally set thirty days as the limit for reimbursable inpatient treatment. They're therefore not designed to provide individualized extended treatment, particularly because of limited resources and lack of an appropriate peer group for the patient who is at Week Six and now repeating much of what was offered during Weeks One through Four. Secondly, the standard four-week program can't provide a person with the gradual increments of freedom and self-direction offered in the extended programs through halfway houses and work programs.

Aftercare

This word is a rather unfortunate one. It sounds rather like "afterthought" and for all too many residential programs is considered little more than that. Insurance may pay for residential treatment, but post-discharge outpatient follow-up and family treatment sessions usually aren't covered. Therefore some aftercare programs are skimpy and short-term. Outpatient group and/or individual therapy should begin promptly after residential treatment and, depending on the recommendations of the treatment team and what's available in your geographical area, may initially be attended as often as several times per week.

Appendix B

Treatment/Rehabilitation Contracts

Sample 1

Tennessee Nurse's Foundation
Peer Assistance Program for Chemically Dependent Nurses

Treatment Contract*

The Peer Assistance Program for Chemically Dependent Nurses, sponsored by the Tennessee Nurse's Foundation and Douglas Arrington, R.N., agree that the following conditions will be fulfilled consistently, truthfully, and with documentation in order that __(Name)__ be maintained in the Peer Assistance Program, thus receiving the protection and support of said program.

1. Will receive treatment for chemical dependence at _____ and will follow all recommendations regarding additional treatment and/or aftercare made by said treatment center.
2. Will contact the Nurse Advocate every Monday.
3. If a relapse should occur while in the PAP, a more extensive healthcare professionals' treatment program will be required. This will include both inpatient and halfway house placement.
4. Will not be involved in the administration of any scheduled medication for the next 12 months.

If __(Name)__ does not comply with the above, the Tennessee Board of Nursing will be notified and the support of the PAP program will be lost. This contract will be reviewed and renegotiated after a period of _____ months, on _____ .

_____   _____
Nurse's Signature   Douglas Arrington, R.N.

*This contract is individualized for each participant.

For further information contact:
Douglas Arrington, R.N.
Tennessee Nurse's Foundation Peer Assistance Program
1720 West End Building, Suite 400
Nashville, Tennessee 37203
(615) 321-0455

Sample 1a
Treatment Contract

Tennessee Nurse's Foundation
Peer Assistance Program for Chemically Dependent Nurses

Release of Information

I, _____ , give permission for _____
      (client)   (TNF confronter)
to release information (written or oral) to _____
concerning my treatment for chemical dependence and participation in the
Tennessee Nurse's Foundation Peer Assistance Program. I understand that
this may include periodic reports as requested. This release is good for the
period I am involved with and followed by the TNF Peer Assistance Program.
I may cancel this release at any time.

I understand that neither the Tennessee Nurse's Foundation Peer Assistance
Program nor any Confronter has control over any action taken as a result of
these reports.

_____   Signature _____
Date   (client)

_____   Signature _____
Date   (confronter)

For further information contact:
Douglas Arrington, R.N.
Tennessee Nurse's Foundation Peer Assistance Program
1720 West End Building, Suite 400
Nashville, Tennessee 37203
(615) 321-0455

Sample 2

Florida Lawyers Assistance, Inc. (F.L.A.)

Description of Advocacy Contract
Based on Operations Manual, Florida Lawyers Assistance, Inc.

The Monitored Rehabilitation Contract is basic to F.L.A.'s operation. It is contructed by F.L.A. staff, agreed to by the attorney and monitored by the Hotline volunteers. It is the document F.L.A. uses to evaluate compliance with the terms of probation, etc. Most importantly, it can serve as a reference and as a path to recovery for the suffering addict. Inadequate as it undoubtedly is, it's F.L.A.'s basic tool.

F.L.A. will normally require an objective professional evaluation prior to constructing a final Rehabilitation Contract unless from the initial personal interview the staff attorney determines that:
1. Attorney admits to alcohol/other drug problem, and
2. Expresses a willingness to accept F.L.A.'s assistance, and
3. By written contract, agrees to pursue rehabilitation in accordance with the contract terms, and
4. Agrees to cooperate with the monitor system, and
5. Agrees to further evaluation and/or treatment in the event of failure of performance, and
6. Alcohol/other drug involvement in charged misconduct is **not** a disputed issue.

Optional Recovery Contracts
Routing Hotline calls involving intervention and/or Hotline contract with caller, resulting in introductions to the Attorney Support Group, Community A.A./N.A. Clubs, etc., are handled without cost reimbursement and in a confidential manner. In these situations, a monitored contract is neither appropriate nor required. However, for
1. Bar applicants with a history of alcohol/other drug use
2. Readmission candidates
3. Attorneys involved in discipline situations
when the call is voluntary, then the call itself, the evaluation, the contract and monitoring, etc., **are and remain confidential.**
However, the attorney is free to disclose F.L.A.'s contract to appropriate bar-related staff, and F.L.A. will testify as the situation requires.

To Care Enough

Mandated Recovery Contracts
1. To carry out Supreme Court Order
    a. Probationary Admissions
    b. Probationary Readmissions
    c. Discipline Probation

2. At the request of appropriate bar staff as a part of ongoing discipline matters
    a. Pre-trial
    b. Pre-sentence
    c. In lieu of continuing the investigation

3. By agreement in minor misconduct cases

Advocacy Contract Guide

Florida Lawyers Assistance, Inc.

Date: _____

1. WHEREAS _____ is an attorney practicing law in _____, Florida, and
2. WHEREAS _____ is an attorney who has been suspended from the practice of law, and
3. WHEREAS _____ is a law student petitioning for Admission to the Florida Bar,
4. WHEREAS _____ has applied for admission to the Florida Bar, and
5. WHEREAS questions have arisen concerning his or her appropriateness to continue said practice, and
6. WHEREAS he or she is considering petitioning for readmission to the Florida Bar, and
7. WHEREAS _____ recognizes a substance abuse problem and desires to attend to his or her rehabilitation,
8. WHEREAS Florida Lawyers Assistance is a Florida corporation organized to assist substance-abusing members of the legal community,
9. WHEREAS Florida Lawyers Assistance has been requested to evaluate his or her alcohol and other drug involvement, evaluate current rehabilitation efforts, and recommend a rehabilitation program,

230

NOW THEREFORE come the parties who agree as follows:

_____(Name)_____ agrees to:

1. Identify an A.A. or N.A. Home Group and attend its weekly meetings.
2. Assist in the organization and growth of an Attorney Support Group in the _____ area.
3. Attend at least 2-3 other A.A. or N.A. meetings per week.
4. Attend 90 A.A. or N.A. meetings in 90 days.
5. After 90 days attend a minimum of three other meetings per week including attorneys' meetings in

   _____.
6. Identify and enlist the aid of an A.A. or N.A. sponsor and give the sponsor permission to disclose appropriate information as requested by Florida Lawyers Assistance.
7. Assume the responsiblity of seeing to it that his or her monitor submit monthly progress reports.
8. Make quarterly phone calls to Charles Hagan, Jr., Executive Director of F.L.A.
9. Secure a copy and read the A.A. or N.A. "Big Book" and the "12 Steps and 12 Traditions."
10. Prepare for and complete the 4th and 5th steps of the A.A. or N.A. 12-Step program within six months.
11. Reimburse the Florida Lawyers Assistance for costs incurred regarding this evaluation and contract in the amount of $200.
12. Reimburse F.L.A. for costs associated with monitoring in the amount of $20 per month. Check payable to F.L.A. and given to monitor and sent with the monthly monitor report.
13. Report to _____ for a 72-96 inpatient evaluation no later than _____.
14. Report to _____ for an evaluation on outpatient basis no later than _____.
15. Renegotiate the terms of this agreement upon receipt of above evaluation.
16. Totally abstain from the use of all mind-altering substances.
17. Encourage spouse to attend Alanon.
18. Encourage his or her_____ to attend Alateen.
19. Discuss the "Guide for the Family" with spouse and encourage participation in the Spouse Support Network.
20. Attend open meetings with spouse if possible.
21. Make restitution as required.

22. Execute an authorization for F.L.A. to secure records from the treatment agencies as required by F.L.A.
23. Carry out his or her aftercare plan as agreed to with the
    _____.
24. Keep an accurate record of A.A. or N.A. meetings and submit an acceptable monthly report to F.L.A.
25. Attend at least _____ Adult Children of Alcoholics meetings.
26. Revise this Contract to include appropriate professional evaluation and/or treatment in the event there is substantial deviation from the terms of this agreement.

Florida Lawyers Assistance agrees to:
1. Provide a phone contact for _____ whenever required.
2. Monitor his or her progress, if required.
3. Provide support through the Attorney's Hotline.
4. Introduce spouse to the Attorney Spouse Support Group.

The client understands and agrees to the following:
1. I understand that strict confidentiality applies until the Florida Bar officials contact F.L.A. concerning the attorney. From **that point on** written authorization to disclose information concerning alcohol and other drug involvement and the rehabilitation therefrom may be executed by the attorney or F.L.A. will continue to hold all prior contracts and information therefrom confidential.
2. I understand that this contract and all information received by F.L.A. pertaining to alcohol and other drug involvement and rehabilitation therefrom will be reported to the appropriate Bar personnel.
3. I will attend the annual meeting and the regional meeting of the Hotline members and clients.

_____   _____
Client   Florida Lawyers Assistance, Inc.

For further information regarding the Florida Lawyers Assistance Program contact:
Charles Hagan, Jr., M.S., J.D.
Executive Director
Florida Lawyers Assistance
5503-A. Pine Island Rd.
Bokeelia, Florida 33922
(813) 283-0088

Sample 3

Pennsylvania Medical Society Impaired Physician Program

Agreement*

I, _____ , agree to the terms of this Agreement between me and the Pennsylvania Medical Society Impaired Physician Program, PMS-IPP, for a period of _____ years beginning on the _____ day of _____, 19 ___, and concluding on the _____ day of _____.

I understand that, if I should not abide by this Agreement, I will release the PMS-IPP from any further advocacy role on my behalf, unless a new Agreement can be reached. I further understand the PMS-IPP will take action as is necessary and/or legally mandated to report my failure to comply with the provisions of this Agreement to persons(s), group(s), or organizations(s) that need to be informed for the sake of investigations, patient protection, and my own well-being and protection. I understand that this Agreement has been designed to allow my colleagues to assist in meeting my personal and professional needs as an impaired physician, and is entered into for the purpose of preventing misunderstanding of the terms and times specified for my participation in the PMS-IPP.

I agree to abide by the following provisions of this agreement:

1. I agree to enter a hospital or treatment center for evaluation, detoxi-fication, and/or rehabilitation or therapy on the_____ day of _____, and will remain until discharged by my therapist(s);
   Facility _____
   Therapist(s) _____

2. I agree to participate in an outpatient rehabilitation or treatment program instead of or following hospitalization for a period of____.
   Facility _____
   Frequency of Therapy _____
   Therapist(s) _____

3. I agree to enter therapy for a period of _____, or until such time as the attending therapist(s)) discharge me from such treatment in collaboration with the PMS-IPP.

* The agreements with PMS-IPP are each individualized to address appropri-ately the particular situation or physician.

(Individual _____; Group _____).
Facility _____
Frequency of Therapy _____
Therapist(s) _____

4. I agree to attend _____ A.A or N.A. meetings per week. I further agree to attend, when available, Caduceus Club meetings, Medical 12-Step Program meetings, and/or other professional recovery group meetings. I will document my attendance and forward a copy monthly to the PMS-IPP. The address of IDAA, International Doctors in A.A., will be forwarded to me for my use in establishing contacts in the recovering physician community.

5. I agree to participate in a specified urine and/or blood analysis program approved by the PMS-IPP.
Frequency of Testing _____
Method _____
Location _____
Monitor _____

6. I agree to seek consultation and evaluation about the usefulness of and indications for the prescription of Antabuse _____ or Naltrexone _____.
Physician/Consultant _____

7. I agree to maintain contact with my PMS-IPP monitor.
Monitor # _____
Frequency of Contact _____

8. I agree to maintain abstinence from the use of any mind-altering drugs (alcohol or other drugs) unless prescribed by another physician in an appropriate manner for an illness with full knowledge and agreement of the PMS-IPP.

9. I agree that my personal physician may inform PMS-IPP of conditions for which I am under treatment including any and all drugs or medications, prescription and over-the-counter, included in the treatment plan. I will also request that drugs of addiction or controlled substances not be prescribed to treat illnesses unless there is no alternative treatment available.

10. I agree to communicate with and/or meet with the Medical Directors of the PMS-IPP periodically to discuss my progress. I further agree to communicate and/or meet with the PMS Committee on the Impaired Physician as deemed necessary.
Frequency of Contact _____

11. I agree to enter into a Contract or Agreement of recovery and relapse consequences with my employer or institution, and give permission for my therapist(s) and the PMS-IPP to communicate with my employer or institution.
Employer(s) _____

_____

For further information contact:
Robert McDermott, M.D.
Greg Gable, M.A.
Pennsylvania Medical Society Impaired Physician Program
20 Erford Road
Lemoyne, Pennsylvania 17043
(717) 763-7937

Sample 4

University of Colorado
Addiction Research and Treatment Services

Memorandum of Agreement

[The following contract is used primarily with professionals who are licensed. It is individualized in the blanks marked PR.]

This is an agreement between **(PR, Name:_____)**, the patient, and Dr. Thomas Crowley to help the patient maintain the resolve to remain free of **(PR, Substance:_____)**. In this agreement the patient directs Dr. Crowley to establish a schedule for collecting urine samples from the patient. **(PR, choose one of the next 3 paragraphs.)**

1. The patient initially will provide urine samples each Monday, Wednesday, and Friday for one month. For the next month Dr. Crowley will prepare a random schedule giving a 67% chance that the patient will be directed to produce a urine sample on any given Monday, Wednesday, or Friday; after the beginning of the third month the random schedule will provide a 33% chance each Monday, Wednesday, and Friday that the patient will be directed to produce a urine sample. The patient will call (355-6176) Dr. Crowley's clinic each Monday, Wednesday, or Friday after the first month to determine whether that is a day for delivering a sample.

2. The patient initially will provide urine samples each Tuesday, Thursday, and Saturday for one month. For the next month Dr. Crowley will prepare a random schedule giving a 67% chance that the patient will be directed to produce a urine sample on any given Tuesday, Thursday, or Saturday; after the beginning of the third month the random schedule will provide a 33% chance each Tuesday, Thursday, or Saturday that the patient will be directed to product a urine sample. The patient will call (355-6176) Dr. Crowley's clinic each Tuesday, Thursday, or Saturday after the first month to determine whether that is a day for delivering a sample.

3. The patient will call (355-6176) Dr. Crowley's clinic every day of the week. The patient will be instructed on each of those days whether he/she is to produce a urine sample on that day. For the first month after signing this agreement, there will be a random 3/7th risk on each day of the week that the patient will be directed to produce a sample. In the second month there will be a 2/7th risk on each day of the week that the patient will be directed to produce a sample. In the third month the risk will decline to 1/7th on each day of the week.

Dr. Crowley or one of his trained employees will observe the urination at Dr. Crowley's clinic at 1827 Gaylord Street, Denver, Colorado. Half of each urine sample will be submitted for analysis at the drug assay laboratory of the Colorado Health Department and half will be saved at Dr. Crowley's clinic. Samples will not be identified by name but only by a code number. Samples will be assayed for **(PR, DRUG:** _____**)**. If the first half of any sample is reported to contain a drug, the second half of that sample will be submitted for a separate analysis.

Most analyses will be done by the Colorado Health Department and will cost an estimated $15.00; rarely, at Dr. Crowley's discretion, gas chromatography or mass spectroscopy analyses costing an estimated $200 may be done in the University of Colorado Department of Pharmacology in a search for unusual drugs. The patient will pay for all analyses.

The patient has supplied Dr. Crowley with a letter and a preaddressed envelope to the Colorado State Board of **(PR, Name of Board:**_____**)** Examiners. This letter states that the patient previously had abused drugs, had entered the present rigorous program of outpatient drug abuse treatment, and that the patient nevertheless resumed drug abuse. In the letter the patient surrenders his or her Colorado **(PR, Kind:**_____**)** license. By this agreement the patient directs Dr. Crowley to mail the letter at any time that both halves of the urine sample are positive for drugs of abuse, or at any time the patient fails to produce a scheduled urine sample.

Each separate analysis requires 1.5 ounces of urine; if the first portion of a sample is positive for drugs, and if the patient has supplied a quantity of urine insufficient for a second analysis, Dr. Crowley is to mail the letter described above. If the quantity is insufficient for even one analysis, that shall be considered a failure of the patient to provide a scheduled sample, and Dr. Crowley is hereby directed to mail the letter as directed above.

If the patient travels out of town, he or she will inform Dr. Crowley in advance of leaving, and the urine collection program will be suspended temporarily during that absence. Dr. Crowley is authorized to verify such absences with **(PR, Name:_____)**. If the patient is sick enough at some time to require hospitalization, Dr. Crowley will arrange another method of collecting urine in the hospital; if the patient is sick and does not require hospitalization, the patient will arrange to produce scheduled urine samples in the usual place. On certain major holidays Dr. Crowley's office and clinic are closed. Dr. Crowley and the patient mutually will agree to altered schedules on these occasions.

If the patient needs, for appropriate medical reasons, one of the drugs to be tested for, he or she will obtain that drug on a legal prescription from a physician or dentist who knows of the patient's drug problem. The patient will supply Dr. Crowley with xeroxed copies of that prescription, and then the appearance of that drug in the urine will not trigger the mailing of the letter. The patient hereby directs Dr. Crowley to communicate by mail or telephone with that prescribing doctor whenever Dr. Crowley deems that communication to be appropriate.

To provide extra surety against mishandling of a urine sample, Dr. Crowley or his assistants will supply the patient with a numbered receipt for each sample, and the patient will double check to assure that the number on the receipt corresponds to the number on the sample bottle. The patient will keep all receipts.

This agreement shall remain in effect for **(PR, Number:_____)** months from the date of signing. If for any reason the patient moves away during the treatment period agreed upon here, and if the patient does not arrange for appropriate follow-up treatment, Dr. Crowley is hereby directed at his discretion to inform the Colorado Board of **(PR, Type of Board:_____)** Examiners that the patient was in treatment with Dr. Crowley for drug abuse, but that the patient prematurely withdrew from that treatment; in this situation Dr. Crowley is **not** to mail the letter which surrenders the patient's license. Dr. Crowley is authorized, under these conditions, to verify with **(PR, Name:_____)** that the patient has moved away from Colorado. During the time of this contract the patient and Dr. Crowley will meet for counseling sessions at a frequency which they will determine.

The patient is strongly encouraged to review this agreement, which may be modified **before** signing, with attorneys, family members, or other advisors. The patient is encouraged to consult an attorney of his or her own choosing regarding the terms of this agreement. He or she may obtain the name of one through the Metropolitan Lawyer Referral Service. Dr. Crowley and the patient agree that this Memorandum of Agreement and the patient's letter to the State Board of (**PR, Type of Board:**_____) Examiners constitute a privileged communication between them, and that a waiver of that privilege shall occur only at the patient's request, or under the terms and conditions stated in this Memorandum of Agreement.

_____   _____
Patient   Doctor

_____   _____
Date   Date

For further information, contact:
Thomas J. Crowley, M.D.
Professor of Psychiatry
Addiction Research and Treatment Services, Executive Director
University of Colorado
Campus Box C 268
4200 E. Ninth Avenue
Denver, Colorado 80262
(303) 394-7573

Appendix C

Monitoring Contracts and Guidelines

Sample 1

Physicians Recovery Network
The Impaired Professionals Program of Florida

Advocacy Contract

_____
Date

Name: _____

Address:_____ (Residence) _____ (Office)

_____   _____

Telephone: _____ (Residence)

_____ (Office)

Specialty: _____

1. I agree to participate in a random urine drug and/or blood screen through (specify by whom and where) _____ within twenty-four hours of notification. I will release by waiver of confidentiality the written results of all such screens to the Physicians Recovery Network to validate my continuing progress in recovery.

    _____ (Initials)

2. I agree to abstain completely from the use of any medications, alcohol, and other mind-altering substances including over-the-counter medica-

241

tions unless ordered by my primary physician, and when appropriate, in consultation with the Physicians Recovery Network.

_____ (Initials)

3. I have selected Dr. _____ as my primary physician located at _____.
   Home telephone # _____ Office telephone #_____
   _____ (Initials)

4. I have selected Dr. _____ as my monitoring physician located at _____.
   Home telephone # _____ Office telephone #_____
   _____ (Initials)

5. I have selected Dr. _____ as supervising physician located at _____.
   Home telephone # _____ Office telephone #_____
   _____ (Initials)

6. I agree to notify the Physicians Recovery Network of any change in address or employment.
   _____ (Initials)

7. I agree to follow the following stipulated conditions concerning my DEA number:_____
   _____ (Initials)

8. I agree to attend a self-help group such as A.A. or N.A. _____ times per week.
   _____ (Initials)

9. I agree to participate in continuing group therapy 1 time per week.
   _____ (Initials)

10. I agree to attend a 12-Step program of professionals in recovery.

_____ (Initials)

11. I agree to notify the Physicians Recovery Network in the event of use of mind-altering substances without a prescription from one of the physicians above.

_____ (Initials)

12. I agree to notify the Physicians Recovery Network by phone or letter 2 times monthly.

_____ (Initials)

13. I agree to provide appropriate release forms for urine or blood screen results, treatment center records, therapist reports and other written and oral information required to comply, and in compliance with the above requests.

_____ (Initials)

14. I agree to withdraw from practice for evaluation at the request of the Physicians Recovery Network if any problem develops.

_____ (Initials)

15. My family will involve themselves in continuing, supportive care.

a) _____ Co-dependence treatment

b) _____ Al-Anon or Naranon

c) _____ Other therapeutic measures (specify)

_____ (Initials)

16. If I fail to comply with this contract it may result in my being reported to DPR through the Physicians Recovery Network.

_____ (Initials)

17. Other requirements

_____.

_____ (Initials)

_____   _____
Witness   Name of Participant   Date

The Physicians Recovery Network agrees to assume an advocacy role with Professional Licensing Board, hospital board, or other appropriate agencies for _____ provided the terms are agreed to and met. The duration of this contract will be for five years with renewal of the case subject to review by the Physicians Recovery Network 60 days prior to the expiration date.

_____   _____
Witness   Physicians Recovery Network   Date

cc: Physicians Recovery Network
      Medical Director, Treatment Program
      Monitoring Physician
      Supervising Physician
      Primary Physician

_____

For further information contact:
Roger Goetz, M.D., Director
Physicians Recovery Network
Florida Medical Foundation
P.O. Box 1881
Fernandina Beach, Florida 32034
(800) 888-8PRN
(904) 277-8004

Sample 2

Florida Lawyers Assistance Program, Inc.

Monitoring Guidelines

In addition to serving as a guide to recovery, the Contract* serves as a basic document for testimony at a formal hearing regarding an attorney's recovery. We must be able to testify that:

1. We evaluated.
2. We formulated a recovery plan.
3. Attorney agreed to its terms in writing.
4. Attorney did or did not peform Contract* obligations.

F.L.A. uses the monitor system to enable it to comment responsibly regarding #4 above.

F.L.A. would not be able to carry out its responsibility to the attorney, the bar, and the public without a solid core of Hotline attorneys volunteering time as monitors.

The monitor report forms should be completed monthly and sent to the F.L.A. together with the attorney's $20 cost reimbursement check. If the attorney has not had sufficient contact with you to allow you to complete the report responsibly, send it in stating just that. Each contract requires the monitored attorney to: "assume responsibility of seeing to it that his or her monitor submit monthly progress reports to F.L.A."

The form has been simplified for ease of operation and to assure its submission in a timely fashion. The following may help to clarify details and give you a sound basis upon which to report.

1. You have been there and are in recovery process. Now apply your practical experience and know-how. They are the most important tools you have to bring to your assignment. No fancy stuff, just the A.A. principles and practices.

---

* See Contract Appendix B (Sample 2).

2. The attitude of the respondent will tell you a great deal. Open cooperation is the ideal. It signifies that there is nothing to hide and shows pride of accomplishment.

3. The extent of involvement in A.A. or N.A. is an excellent predictor of success or failure.

4. A strong support structure is also very important: certainly, an A.A. or N.A. sponsor and an identified home group, as a minimum. The degree of family support and participation is another factor to determine results of rehabilitation efforts.

5. We do not practice law in a vacuum. The respondent's progress as reflected in remarks of colleagues will often offer clues to rehabilitation progress.

6. Occasionally a condition of probation will specifically order hospital observation, urine screening, psychological consultation, outpatient group therapy, inpatient rehabilitation, and the like. In these cases, arrangements will be made and appropriate provisions included in the rehabilitation contract. However, the rehabilitation contract has not been cast in concrete. Discuss changes or modifications with the Executive Director. It's results we are after.

Sample 2a

Florida Lawyers Assistance Program, Inc.

Monitor's Report

Report covers dates: _____

Name of participant: _____

Approximately how often did you have informal contact and/or opportunity to observe the participant during this period? _____

Comments: _____

Ratings (please rank on scale):

Attitude _____

	0	1	2	3	4	5
	Negative				Cooperative/Positive	

Compliance with treatment plan:

	0	1	2	3	4	5
	Poor					Excellent

Compliance with monitor plan:

	0	1	2	3	4	5
	Poor					Excellent

Functioning in legal setting:

	0	1	2	3	4	5
	Poor					Excellent

Functioning in other areas:

0	1	2	3	4	5

Poor   Excellent

Comments (please explain any low ratings, any recommendations you might have, etc.):

_____

Monitor

_____

Date

For further information contact:
Charles Hagan, Jr., M.S., J.D., Executive Director
Florida Lawyers Assistance
5503-A. Pine Island Rd.
Bokeelia, Florida 33922
(813) 283-0088

Sample 3

*California Medical Association Guidelines**
for Monitoring a Physician for Chemical Dependence
by the Medical Staff

The purpose of monitoring is to assure the medical staff that a physician with patient care responsibilities can practice medicine safely.

The medical staff must be satisfied that the physician's current health and mental health meet the medical staff's standards of appointment, reappointment, or resumption of patient care.

The medical staff must acknowledge that ongoing consistent monitoring is required for a specified period of time (a minimum of two years), and sufficient resources of physician time and attention must be allocated for it.

1. A Monitoring Plan: A Monitoring Agreement
   A monitoring plan should be drawn up, and it should serve as the basis of a monitoring agreement between the designated medical staff committee and the physician. The following elements should be addressed as the plan is designed:

   A. Treatment
   The medical staff committee should satisfy itself that the physician receives appropriate treatment sufficient to ensure that the problem is being addressed effectively. The medical staff committee should satisfy itself that the physician's current health and mental health are sufficient to allow him or her to practice safely.

   An initial course of treatment appropriate to the situation should be instituted and completed.

   The monitoring plan should incorporate the elements of an aftercare plan and recovery plan which have been recommended by those responsible for initial treatment.

* Excerpt from Guidelines.

249

B. Release of Information

The medical staff committee should require that the physician authorize the therapist(s) to communicate information to the medical staff
committee. Information should come from those responsible for primary care (initial treatment) as well as aftercare and/or ongoing care.

C. Recovery Plan

The physician should have a specific, ongoing recovery plan sufficient
to the situation and to the physician's status in recovery. The monitoring plan should be designed to accumulate the information which will,
over time, document the physician's participation in this recovery
program.

Regular participation in a self-help group of persons in recovery from
chemical dependence (where appropriate, a group of physicians or
health professionals in recovery) should be required.

D. Information to Be Gathered and Reviewed

Information about the health status of the physician in recovery and
about his or her performance should be gathered and reviewed. The
process of gathering and evaluating such information is called monitoring. Information should come from several sources appropriate to the
physician's situation, such as:

—from the hospital workplace
—from body fluid test results
—from an aftercare coordinator
—from ongoing therapist
—from family
—from office colleagues

The medical staff committee should designate those who are in a
position to gather and submit to the coordinator of monitoring the
different kinds of information appropriate to the case. These monitors
should be appointed as members of the medical staff committee for the
purpose of carrying out this activity so that the peer review protections
will be applicable.

E. Regular Contact with a Knowledgeable Observer

There should be a regular, face-to-face contact between the physician and a monitor knowledgeable about chemical dependence and about what to look for in a physician with the condition of being monitored. The time and place of the contact should vary. The frequency and length of contact should be determined for each case. For some, daily or even more than once-a-day contact may be indicated, especially in the first days or weeks of the monitoring process. Most usually, three times a week would be considered a minimum for the initial period. The frequency would vary with the particular physician's status in recovery. The length of contact must be sufficient to make an observation of the physician's behavior. The record should include periodic notes based on this observation. The monitors should be able to create a relationship of mutual trust, support, helpfulness, and respect. Monitors, however, should maintain objectivity and diligence throughout the monitoring process.

F. Coordinator of Monitoring

All who serve as sources of information should report to one coordinator of monitoring for the case, and that person should be a member of the hospital staff committee. The function of the coordinator is to assemble all the information and to review, interpret, evaluate, and respond to the comprehensive picture.

G. Body Fluid Testing

Body fluid testing is desirable as one element of a monitoring plan. Body fluids (most commonly urine) should be collected on a random schedule and under direct observation.

NOTE: Body fluid testing alone does not comprise a sufficient monitoring plan and is not the highest priority element of the plan. Greater weight is given to regular observation of behavior by a knowledgeable monitor. The monitoring agreement should specify what role body fluid testing will have in the overall monitoring plan. Where body fluid testing is required, the test done must be able to detect the drug(s) which the physician might use. The agreement should describe how positive results will be interpreted and what will be the response of the medical staff committee to positive results. The monitoring agreement should specify the costs of testing and who pays the cost. The results should be sent to the coordinator of monitoring.

H. Regular Conferences

There should be a mechanism for face-to-face conferences at the request of any of these parties, between the monitors, the physician monitored, the coordinator of monitoring, and the medical staff committee responsible for the monitoring.

I. Reevaluation of the Recovery Plan and the Monitoring Plan

There should be regular reevaluation at some interval, perhaps every six months, of the monitoring plan by the medical staff committee to assure that it is sufficient to the need but does not require elements no longer necessary to the situation. Changes in the plan should be made so that it fits the current situation of the physician and his/her status in recovery. It may or may not be appropriate to have this evaluation made by an acknowledged expert outside of the medical staff who will provide a written report. The monitoring agreement should specify the cost of this evaluation and who pays the cost.

J. Record Keeping

For each case where there is monitoring, there must be a record. The record should include a copy of the signed monitoring agreement between the physician and the committee. The medical staff committee must have adequate information to assess the physician's status in recovery and compliance with the elements in the agreement. This information must be accumulated in the record and must be kept in strict confidence, preferably in a locked file or other secure storage which may be accessed only by committee members. This information should be retained indefinitely, preferably as long as the physician practices in the hospital plus five years. Disclosure of this information outside the committee should be made only at the written request of the individual involved or with the advice of legal counsel.

K. Response to "Slips"

The monitoring plan should take into consideration the fact that a relapse or resumption of use of alcohol or other drugs (or a "slip") is not an uncommon phenomenon for those in recovery from chemical dependence, especially in the early phases of recovery. Statistics show that slips occur in a significant percent of cases, usually within the first year of sobriety. The response to a slip should be the same as a response to the initial diagnosis; that is, the slip should be assessed by a knowledgeable, experienced evaluator, and the response should be tailored to the situation.

A slip alone should not be considered cause for termination of privileges or loss of employment or position. The customary response to a slip is to intensify the treatment plan, of which monitoring is a part, for a period of time appropriate to the case. It may or may not be appropriate to require that the physician take a leave from patient care for a period of time appropriate to the situation. Consideration should be given to the physician's health and to patient safety in reaching a decision about whether a leave is appropriate.

For further information contact:
Fern Leger
California Medical Association
221 Main Street, P.O. Box 7690
San Francisco, California 94120-7690
(415) 541-0900

Appendix D

Return-to-Work Contracts

Sample 1

*N.U.R.S.E.S. of Colorado Corporation**

Return-to-Work Agreement

Name of Institution :

_____

Nurse Employee: _____

Date: _____   19___

This Agreement is to clarify expectations regarding the return to work of
_____ (nurse) and _____ (employer).

This Agreement shall be in effect from _____, 19 ____, to _____, 19___.
The contents of this Agreement are mutually agreed upon and may be
modified quarterly as deemed necessary and agreed upon by both parties.
Work attendance and job performance will be monitored closely.

I, _____, RN/LPN agree to:

1. Abstain from mind-altering drugs, alcohol and/or potentially addicting
   medications. In the event that such medications may be needed as a part
   of my health care, I agree to notify my employer, _____
   _____, immediately. This must be documented
   by a prescription. Over-the-counter drugs must also be reported prior
   to use.

* This agreement should be tailored to your individual employment setting.

2. Participate in an aftercare program as recommended by my treatment provider, _____. Therapist name: _____. Aftercare plan attached.
3. Provide random urines for _____ year(s) on a (weekly) (bimonthly) (monthly) basis. These will be monitored, collected, and reported by _____ to (employer designee) _____.
   Urine screens will be paid for by (employee) (employer) _____.
   Should a narcotic discrepancy occur on my shift on my unit, I agree to submit a urine sample for testing.
4. Cooperate with supervision regarding narcotic sign-out and charting for _____ months. (In cases where narcotic addiction is involved, it is recommended that narcotic administration **not** be a responsibility of the recovering nurse or employee for one year.)
5. Work with N.U.R.S.E.S. of Colorado Corporation peer employee assistance program for a minimum of twelve months. I agree to sign a Professional Monitoring Agreement with N.U.R.S.E.S. of Colorado Corporation.
6. Attend _____ A.A. or N.A. meetings per week for_____ months. Attendance will be agreed upon between myself and my therapist or counselor and this agreement communicated to the employer designee, _____.

The undersigned agree to determine modifications in the employment setting in order to support the nurse's recovery process. These modifications shall include but not be limited to the following:
Assigned unit, shift, and supervision
Administration of narcotics
Possession of narcotics key
Time off for A.A. or N.A. aftercare or peer support meetings
Use of buddy system

This agreeement and all the conditions therein shall remain confidential.

_____   _____
Employee   Date

_____   _____
Nurse Manager   Date

_____   _____
Occupational Health Nurse   Date

_____   _____
                                              Date

_____
For further information contact:
Elizabeth M. Pace, B.S., R.N., C.E.A.P.
N.U.R.S.E.S. of Colorado Corporation
P.O. Box 61294
Denver, Colorado 80206
(303) 758-0596 (24-hour answering service)

Sample 2

Nurse Recovery Program
Tampa Area Hospital Council

Return-to-Work Contract (Description, Procedure)

Description

The purpose of the Return-to-Work Contract is to assist the employer and the nurse in clear understanding of regulatory, treatment, and employer guidelines for nurses enrolled in the Nurse Recovery Program. It is recommended that this contract be initiated for each nurse who has been identified through the Nurse Recovery Program, has received treatment, and is returning to the workplace.

Procedure

1. Ideally the contract should be completed prior to the time of returning to work.

2. A meeting may be scheduled with the nursing employee, nursing executive/ and or personnel director, head nurse, and Nurse Recovery Program liaison approximately one week prior to the time the nurse will be returning to the work setting.

3 It is recommended that prior to this meeting the individuals have in writing the treatment recommendations and aftercare plan from the treatment center in order to facilitate development of this contract.

4. Once this contract has been completed it is recommended that copies be sent to each of the individuals who have signed the contract, including the liaison for the Nurse Recovery Program. This is to be maintained in the nurse's file.

5. This return-to-work contract has been devised as a guideline; certainly other pertinent information may be added according to individual need.

Return-to-Work Contract

It is the purpose of this contract to protect you, the employee, and to protect the hospital from any misunderstanding as to the terms of your return to work. This contract is specifically designed to meet the needs of both the individual and the institution.

1. I, _____, agree to the terms of this contract for a period of two years from the date of this contract. I understand that failure to comply with the terms of this contract may result in immediate termination.

2. I understand that all expenses connected with my treatment or rehabilitation are to be rendered at my own expense and are my own responsibility.

3. I agree to a rehabilitation program which will consist of :

   a) Attendance at regular A.A. and/or N.A. meetings no less frequently than _____ times per week. I agree to furnish documentation of attendance to _____ on a weekly basis.

   b) Attendance once a week at a Recovering Nurse Support Group sponsored by the Tampa Area Hospital Council's Nurse Recovery Program. I agree to furnish documentation of attendance at such meetings to _____ on a weekly basis.

   c) Continuation of my therapy with _____ until such time as I am released from treatment. I agree to provide documentation of my release to _____.

4. I hereby authorize my therapist to contact and exchange information regarding my progress with _____.

5. I hereby authorize _____ to contact and exchange information pertaining to my treatment with _____ for the following purposes: _____
   _____.

6. I agree to completely abstain from any mind-altering chemicals (alcohol, sedatives, stimulants, narcotics, soporifics, over-the-counter drugs, etc.) except as recommended by my physician and with approval of my counselor or Nurse Recovery Program.

7. I agree to provide random urine and blood samples in the presence of a qualified witness at the discretion of my nurse manager. I understand that I will be responsible for the cost of these monitoring measures.

8. I will follow the treatment as recommended by those managing my care. I understand that if I do not comply with the treatment it could mean the loss of my employment.

9. Other:

_____

Employee Signature   Date

_____

Personnel Signature   Date

_____

Nursing Administrator/Designee   Date

_____

Director, Nurse Recovery Program   Date

cc: Employee
       Personnel
       Nursing Administrator
       Nurse Recovery Program
_____

For information contact:
Linda R. Crosby, M.S.N., R.N.
130 Federal St., #3
Salem, MA 01970
(508) 744-2162

Appendix E

Relapse Guidelines

Nurse Recovery Program
Tampa Area Hospital Council

Relapse Policy

As is stated in the philosophy of the Nurse Recovery Program, we understand and accept that alcohol/other drug addiction is a disease. One of the critical components of this disease is relapse, which is an inherent risk in each person who has been diagnosed as chemically dependent. Because nurses are licensed personnel, responsible for rendering care to the consumers in our hospitals, we maintain that relapse is a potentially serious occurrence and must be individually evaluated. The policy of the Nurse Recovery Program for a relapse of any person enrolled in the program is as follows:

1. The nurse will report the relapse to her or his counselor, supervisor, or Nurse Recovery Program.

2. The relapse may be identified in the workplace or in aftercare or by the Nurse Recovery Program.

3. Once identified and/or reported, the nurse will be evaluated by a treatment team initially comprised of her or his aftercare counselor, the medical director for the treatment program in which the nurse was treated, a nurse liaison, and the director of the Nurse Recovery Program and/or designees of the nursing administrator. The nurse will be removed from duty pending this evaluation and/or assessment.

4. If the treatment team cannot come to a resolution regarding recommendations for the treatment for this nurse, or if there is a clinical question not resolved at this meeting, the nurse may be requested to submit to evaluation by the Medical Advisory Committee of the Nurse Recovery Program for individual assessment, evaluation, and treatment recommendations.

5. After this/these evaluation(s) a meeting will be held with the nurse, the director of the Nurse Recovery Program, treating professionals, and/or nursing administrator or designee. An outline of the recommended treatment/restructuring of the recovery program will be presented to the nurse.

6. The Impaired Nurse Program (sponsored by the Board of Nursing) will be advised of all the above steps as they are taken with the person who participates in that program.

7. The Nurse Recovery Program reserves the right to discharge from the program any nurse who has not complied with the treatment recommendations made by the treating professionals and/or with recommendations made by the participating hospital (employer).

For further information contact:
Linda R. Crosby, M.S.N., R.N.
130 Federal St., #3
Salem, MA 01970
(508) 744-2162

Appendix F

Laboratory Testing for Mind-Altering Drugs

Proper use of random drug screening, whether of urine or blood, requires selection of laboratory services that provide a variety of levels of testing; protocols for confirmation of positive results; oral and hard-copy reporting procedures; expertise in chain-of-custody and confidentiality procedures; and availability of expert medical consultation on problematic issues of drug screening.

It's advisable to assess the laboratory's experience and expertise in drug screening by meeting with a representative and exploring all related issues of concern.

Laboratory Methods of Urine Drug Screen Testing

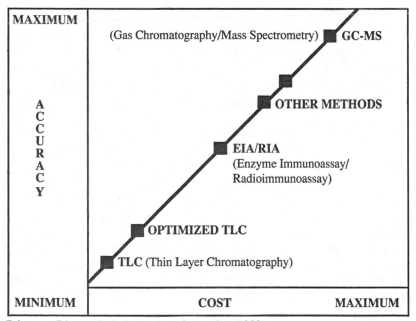

Princeton Diagnostic Laboratories of America (1988)

263

Types of Testing Available

1. Thin Layer Chromatography (TLC) is one of the oldest drug-screening methods. It has great sensitivity for detecting many substances but is time-consuming and requires well-developed technical expertise in the person who interprets results. The reliability of the TLC therefore depends on the person who interprets the findings; this decreases its effectiveness as a primary screening method. The TLC may also be affected by use of over-the-counter preparations and some medications. The TLC is popular as a confirmatory test when positive results are obtained by another testing method.

2. Enzyme Immunoassay (EIA) is another currently popular drug-screening method. It includes Enzyme-Multipled Immunoassay Technique (EMIT). The immunoassay test displays the reaction between a specific testing substance or antibody and the specific drug with which it has reacted. The EMIT method can detect the presence of over 35 drugs, including amphetamines, barbiturates, benzodiazepines, opiates, and marijuana, cocaine, methadone, PCP, Darvon, and Quaaludes.

This method of screening is highly sensitive and widely used as a standard screening method for monitoring or for documenting suspicion of drug use in cases where employee intervention is initiated. However, the EMIT's sensitivity does create a cross-reaction with other drugs in the same classification that have a similar chemical structure and sometimes misreads the actual drug. As with the TLC screening, some over-the-counter preparations can interfere with accurate identification of drugs present. Positive results are confirmed through another method that will validate the drug present and the amount.

Other immunoassay methods of testing may be used, but the EMIT profile provides the most comprehensive screening method available at a moderate cost.

3. Gas Chromatography and Mass Spectrometry (GC/MS), known as GC Mas Spec. to those in the field, is the most accurate test available to confirm both the presence of a particular drug and the actual amount present. It's the most reliable method of confirmation and should be routinely ordered when a positive screening result is obtained on a professional in recovery. Obtaining this method of confirmation documents with maximum assurance the presence of even very minute amounts of the drug in question. The GC/MS is expensive, but when absolute confirmation is required the cost becomes secondary. This test can also provide confirmation of the **absence** of a drug that may have been reported on primary screening and can reassure those who are monitoring the professional that the first report was a "false positive."

Certain substances such as high concentrations of over-the-counter products or even the ingestion of certain foods in large quantities may on rare occasions affect the results of the screening, and, although the person has not relapsed, a positive urine may be reported.

In selecting laboratory services it's wise to request that any specimens from your program that test positive be confirmed by GC/MS automatically rather than by standard laboratory confirmation methods. This procedure will assure you that there either definitely **is** a problem or that the first testing was a false positive. In cases where we may need to initiate action based on the laboratory results, the GC/MS will provide accurate, reliable documentation.

Limits of Detection

It's important to understand that most laboratory screening methods are limited in their ability to detect drugs that are present in only minute quantities. Each laboratory has an established concentration limit that must be met for each drug in order for the testing to identify its presence. Some drugs, for example, are broken down quickly in the body and excreted in the urine, and although the subject may have taken a particular drug, the quantity left in the urine isn't enough to trigger a positive response on the testing.

Similarly, laboratories have defined cutoff limits for what is called **positive** and what is called **negative**. These limits are essentially based on the limits of detection for the specific testing methods used and reduce the probability of reporting inaccurate information. For example, if the cutoff limit for marijuana is 50, that means that marijuana may be present but that if it's under 50 lab measures it's regarded as negative (passive inhalation of marijuana has been known to show in small quantities in the urine). The limits for positive and negative have been established on the basis of significant research and experience and ultimately provide the most reliable results for the presence of each specific drug, but what they don't tell us is when and how the drug was used. Of course the purpose of monitoring is to detect if any drugs were used, rather than to document impairment.

Another factor that complicates the process of urine screening in recovery is that as the period between the use of the drug and the actual testing lengthens, the probability becomes greater that the testing may not document the use. So getting a urine sample as quickly as possible from a suspected professional is imperative if positive results are to be used as leverage.

Approximate Retention Time of Drugs in the Urine*

Drug	Approximate Retention Time
Amphetamines	1-2 days
Barbiturates	
1. Short-acting (Nembutal, Seconal, Seral	1-3 days
2. Long-acting (Phenobarbital, Mebaral)	1-3 weeks
Benzodiazepines (Xanax, Librium, Tranxene, Dalmane, Valium, Serax, etc.)	1-14 days
Cannabinoids (marijuana by-products)	Occasional use, 1-7 days Chronic use, 1-4 weeks
Cocaine metabolites	12-48 hours
Opiates (Demerol, Dilaudid, Morphine, Stadol, Talwin, Fentanyl)	1-3 days

*Smith Kline Bio-Science Laboratories, 1987. Names of specific mind-altering drugs added by authors.

A similar problem is that when screening methods such as the EMIT are used, the test will report only on those specific drugs, but if the person has other drugs present in the urine, they won't be reported unless the test is specifically designed to identify them. So a negative EMIT screening indicates that none of the drugs on the assay is present, but there may be something else present that wasn't tested.

Considerations in Selecting a Laboratory

1. What type of testing does it usually perform?
2. How does it confirm a positive result?
3. What methods does it use in reporting?

4. What's the usual turn-around time?
5. How long does it retain specimens?
6. Does it have a consultant available to discuss problems and concerns?

Procedure for Positive Results

1. **Don't panic.** Laboratory errors are common. Also, depending on the type of testing you select, there may be a higher incidence of "false positives." There are many interactions of medications, even food by-products, that interfere with some testing methods.
2. **Have the lab send a specimen for GC/MS confirmation.** This is drug-specific and will identify the presence of a particular drug to the tenth of a nanogram.
3. **Request another specimen from the employee.** Follow the same "observed urine procedure" and chain-of-custody procedures as given in Chapter 8.
4. **Send a second specimen for RIA testing.** Also, request confirmation of any positives with GC/MS.

Appendix G

Selected Resources

Books

Aguilera, D., and J. Messick. *Crisis Intervention: Theory and Methodology*. St. Louis: The C.V. Mosby Company, 1978.

Bissell, L., and P. Haberman. *Alcoholism in the Professions*. New York: Oxford University Press, 1984.

Bissell, L., and J. Royce. *Ethics for Addiction Professionals*. Center City, Minn.: Hazelden Foundation, 1987.

Brown, S. *Treating the Alcoholic*. New York: John Wiley and Sons, 1985.

Dogoloff, L., and R. Angarola. *Urine Testing in the Workplace*. New York: American Council for Drug Education, 1985.

Johnson Institute Books. *How to Use Intervention in Your Professional Practice*. Minneapolis, 1987.

Johnson, V. *I'll Quit Tomorrow*. San Francisco: Harper & Row, 1980.

Johnson, V. *Intervention: How to Help Someone Who Doesn't Want Help*. Minneapolis: Johnson Institute Books, 1986.

Robertson, N. *Getting Better: Inside Alcoholics Anonymous*. New York: William Morrow, 1988.

Schwebel, M., J. Skorina, and G. Schoener. *Assisting Impaired Psychologists*. Washington, D.C.: American Psychological Association, 1988.

Sullivan, E.J., L. Bissell, and E. Williams. *Chemical Dependency in Nursing: The Deadly Diversion*. Redwood City, Cal.: Addison-Wesley Publishing Co., 1987.

Booklets

Bissell, L. *Some Perspectives on Alcoholism.* Minneapolis: Johnson Institute.

Johnson Institute Books.*The Family Enablers*, revised edition. Minneapolis: Johnson Institute, 1987.

Articles

American Medical Association Council on Scientific Affairs. "Issues in Employee Drug Testing." *Journal of the American Medical Association* 258, no. 15 (Oct.16, 1987): 2089-96.

American Medical Association Council on Scientific Affairs. "Scientific Issues in Drug Testing. " *Journal of the American Medical Association* 257, no. 22 (June 12, 1987): 3110-14.

Bissell, L., and J. Skorina. "One Hundred Alcoholic Women in Medicine." *Journal of the American Medical Association* 257, no. 21 (June 5, 1987): 2939-44.

Bissell, L., and R. W. Williams. "Pharmacists Recovering from Alcoholism." *American Pharmacist.* June 1989 (in press).

Shea, P. "Drug and Alcohol Testing in the Workplace: Passing the Legal Test." *Clinical Laboratory Management Review,* Jan. 1987, 23-29.

Videos

Back to Reality
Johnson Institute (1989)
7151 Metro Boulevard
Minneapolis, MN 55435
(800) 231-5165

Chemical Dependency in Nursing
Gary Whiteaker Corporation (1989)
109 A West Washington
Millstadt, IL 62260
(618) 476-7771

Enabling: Masking Reality
Johnson Institute (1989)
7151 Metro Boulevard
Minneapolis, MN 55435
(800) 231-5165

Impaired Nursing Practice
American Journal of Nursing
Company
555 West 57th Street
New York, NY 10019-2961
(212) 582-8820

Intervention: Facing Reality
Johnson Institute (1989)
7151 Metro Boulevard
Minneapolis, MN 55435
(800) 231-5165

Appendix H

Resources for Professional Information, Programs, Groups

National Information Centers on Chemical Dependence

National Institute on Alcohol Abuse and Alcoholism (NIAAA), 5600 Fishers Lane, Rockville, MD 20857

National Institute on Drug Abuse (NIDA), 5600 Fishers Lane, Rockville, MD 20857

National Council on Alcohol, 12 W. 21st Street, New York, NY 10010; (212) 206-6770

Professional Organizations Providing Information and Assistance

Many of the following also know of mutual support groups and provide contacts for networking with professionals in recovery.

American Academy of Physician Assistants
Sub-Committee on Impaired Practitioners
950 N. Washington Street
Alexandria, VA 22314
(703) 836-AAPA

American Bar Association
Commission on Impaired Lawyers
750 Lakeshore Drive
Chicago, IL 60611
(312) 988-5345
Contact: Roseanne Theis

American Dental Association
Council on Dental Practice
211 E. Chicago Avenue
Chicago, IL 60611
(312) 440-2622
Contact : William Oberg

American Judicature Society
25 E. Washington Street, Suite 1600
Chicago, IL 60602
(312) 558-6900
Contact: Kate Sampson

American Medical Association
Department of Substance Abuse/Physician Assistance Program
535 Dearborn Street
Chicago, IL 60610
(312) 645-5079
Contact: Janice Robertson

American Medical Society on Alcoholism and Other Addictions
12 W. 21st Street
New York, NY 10010
(212) 206-6770

American Medical Women's Association
Impaired Physician Committee
801 N. Fairfax Street
Alexandria, VA 22314
(703) 838-0500
Contact: Eileen McGrath, J.D.

American Nurses Association
2420 Pershing Road
Kansas City, MO 64108
(816) 474-5720
Contact: Staff person assigned to
Committee on Impaired Nursing Practice

American Osteopathic Association
Membership Department
142 E. Ontario Street
Chicago, IL 60611
(800) 621-1773

American Pharmaceutical Association
2215 Constitution Avenue, NW
Washington, D.C. 20037
(202) 429-7532
Contact: Ronald Williams, R.Ph.

American Podiatric Medical Association
Committee for the Rehabilitation of Impaired Podiatrists
9312 Old Georgetown Road
Bethesda, MD 20814
(301) 571-9200
Hotline: (407) 352-9666

American Psychiatric Association
Office of Education
1400 K Street, NW
Washington, D.C. 20005
(202) 682-6130
Contact: Staff representative for
Committee on the Impaired Physician

American Psychological Association
Committee on Impaired Psychologists
1200 17th Street, NW
Washington, D.C. 20036
(202) 955-7644
Contact: Sheila Lane-Forsyth

American Veterinary Medical Association
930 N. Meacham Road
Schaumburg, IL 60196
(800) 248-2862 (answering machine 24 hours)
Contact: Joe Gloyd

Association of Labor-Management Administrators
and Consultants to Alcoholism (ALMACA)
1800 N. Kent Street, Suite 907
Arlington, VA 22209
(703) 522-6272

Drug and Alcohol Nursing Association (DANA)
113 W. Franklin Street
Baltimore, MD 21201
(301) 752-3318

National Association of Social Workers (NASW)
7981 Eastern Avenue
Silver Spring, MD 20910
(800) 638-8799
(301) 565-0333
Contact: Norma J. Taylor, Ph.D.

National Catholic Council on Alcoholism
and Related Drug Problems
1200 Varnum Street, NE
Washington, D.C. 20017-2796
(202) 832-3811
Contact: Reverend John F.X. O'Neill

National Nurses Society on Addictions (NNSA)
2500 Gross Point Road
Evanston, IL 60201
(312) 475-7530

Canada

Canadian Medical Association
Department of Health Services/Physicians at Risk
1867 Alta Vista Drive
Ottawa, Canada K1G068
(613) 731-9331

Mutual Help and Networking Groups

Al-Anon Family Groups
P.O. Box 862, Midtown Station
New York, NY 10018-0862
(212) 302-7240

Alcoholics Anonymous (A.A.)
P.O. Box 459, Grand Central Station
New York, NY 10163
(212) 686-1100

Cocaine Anonymous (C.A.)
P.O. Box 1367
Culver City, CA 90232
(213) 559-5833

Narcotics Anonymous (N.A.)
P.O. Box 9999
Van Nuys, CA 91409
(818) 780-3951

Mutual Support Groups for Professionals

Anesthetists in Recovery (AIR)
3413 Sailmaker Lane
Plano, TX 75023
(214) 369-4111 (O)
(214) 596-5382 (H)
Contact: Beth Visintine, C.R.N.A.

Intercongregational Alcoholism Program (ICAP)
1921 N. Harlem Avenue, #104
Chicago, IL 60635-3792
(312) 637-1656
Contacts: Letitia Close, B.V.M., C.A.C., or Mary Gene Kinney, B.V.M., C.A.C.
Open to sisters and former sisters who are members of A.A. or Al-Anon, or who are working in the chemical dependence field. Most members are educators, but quite a few are members of nursing orders.

International Doctors in A.A. (IDAA)
P.O. Box 444
Center City, MN 55012
(612) 835-4421 (O)
(612) 929-6123 (H)
Contact: C. Richard McKinley, M.D.
Open to any doctoral-level healthcare professional or matriculated student in a program leading to a doctoral degree. Al-Anon doctors welcome. Members include M.D., D. O., D.V.M., D.S.W., Ph.D. or Ed.D. in psychology, nursing, medical science.

International Lawyers in A.A. (ILAA)
1092 Elm Street, Suite 201
Rocky Hill, CT 06067
(203) 529-7474
Contact: Igor I. Sikorsky, Jr.
Open to attorneys and law students in recovery from chemical dependence.

International Nurses Anonymous
1020 Sunset Drive
Lawrence, KS 66044
(913) 842-3893
Pat Green, R.N., M.S.W.
Open to nurses who are in personal recovery or who are members of Al-Anon.

International Pharmacists Anonymous
36 Cedar Grove Road
Annandale, NJ 08801
(201) 730-9072 (H)
Contact: Nan Davis, Listkeeper

Open to all pharmacists and pharmacy students who are members of recovery programs or considering that they might belong in one.

The JACS Foundation
197 E. Broadway
Room M-7 at the Educational Alliance
New York, NY 10002
(212) 473-4747
Open membership. Sponsors retreat weekends for Jewish chemical dependents in recovery and their families. Active in community professional education about chemical dependence. Many of its members are healthcare professionals, and most are in recovery programs.

National Association of Lesbian and Gay
Alcoholism Professionals (NALGAP)
108 Fuller Street
Brookline, MA 02140
(617) 736-5146 (H)
Contact: Fraelean Curtis, L.I.C.S.W.
or
NALGAP
204 W. 20th Street
New York, NY 10011
(212) 713-5074
No membership requirements but does have very modest membership fee. Members include all healthcare disciplines, some clergy and attorneys. Most are gay or lesbian or family members. Most are members of 12-Step programs and/or working in the chemical dependence field. Can provide support, information, and networking for those who are concerned about issues of sexual orientation.

Physician Assistants
University Health Service
University of Michigan
207 Fletcher Street
Ann Arbor, MI 48109-1050
(313) 764-2080
Contact: Lyn Hadley, R.N., PA-C

Psychologists Helping Psychologists
23439 Michigan Ave.
Dearborn, MI 48124
(313) 565-3821
Contact: Jane Skorina, Ph.D.
Open to doctoral-level psychologists who are chemical dependents in recovery.

Social Workers Helping Social Workers
South Street
Goshen, CT 06756
(203) 491-3309
Contact: John Fitzgerald, M.S.W., Ph.D.
or
Lock Box 1133, Grand Central Station
New York, NY 10017
(203) 489-3808
Open to all M.S.W.'s and students currently enrolled in an M.S.W. program who are in personal recovery or who are members of Al-Anon.

There are literally hundreds of mutual-support groups, many of them for chemically dependent people, many others for their friends and families. Some are quite specialized, such as groups for alcoholics with AIDS, or for adult children of alcoholic parents. A complete listing is beyond the scope of this book, but information is available from:

Self-Help Clearinghouse
Saint Clare's-Riverside Medical Center
Denville, NJ 07834
(201) 625-7101, TDD (201) 625-9053
Compu Serve 70275, 1003.

This clearinghouse publishes *The Self-Help Sourcebook*, which lists national offices for most groups that have them and can tell you how to find or, if need be, form local groups to meet almost any specific need. Groups and networks for chemical dependents are available in many countries and in many languages; they include ham radio operators and computer groups. Never assume that there's no group for the very special professional who's trying to convince you he or she is too unique to recover. More than likely the situation isn't unique and a group exists. Assume it's there to be found.

Index

Abscesses, as sign of chemical dependence, 82-83

Absenteeism
documentation of, 82-83
policies for, 44

Abstinence, 18-19, 56

Acceptance phase of grieving, 157-158

Access to drugs by healthcare professionals, 21-23

Action plan development, 103-116, 123
anticipating excuses, 115
crisis situations, 106-109
determining leverage, 104-106
insurance and benefit assessments, 110-111
intervention locale, 109-110
post-intervention transportation arrangements, 114-115
safety precautions, 116
securing evaluation or treatment bed, 111-114
timing of intervention, 106
subject's participation in, 161-162
"what-if" considerations, 117-122

Addiction potential of drugs, 16-17

Administrative personnel. *See* Employer; Management

Administrator on intervention team, 126, 191-192

Advocacy contract, 229-232

Advocacy programs, 64-65

Aftercare, 219, 226
issues of, 192-194
planning, 187-188
relapse and, 211-212

Agreement memorandum, 236-239

Airline industry, alcohol/other drug use in, 56

Alcohol
social acceptability of, 55-56
detecting presence of, 138, 204-205

Alcohol/other drugs
addiction potential of, 16-17
defined, 1
license revocations and disbarments due to, 11
manipulating supply or surroundings, 38
pleasure from, 15-16
relapse with, 212-213

Ambivalence of team members, 170

Anesthesia/surgical records, as intervention data source, 75

Anger phase of grieving, 155-156

Anonymity, treatment center selection and, 113
See also Confidentiality

Authority figure in intervention
"bottom line" statement, 140
recommendations and alternatives from, 139

"Bad guy" role on intervention team, 58-59, 131

Bargaining
grieving during intervention, 156
long-term treatment and, 186-187
by subject during intervention, 152-153

Behavioral changes
as chemical dependence indicator, 79-81
relapses and, 212

Black eyes, chemical dependence indicator, 82

"Blackout", documentation of, 17-18, 81

Blaming, among intervention team, 102

Blood Alcohol Concentration (BAC) test, 204-205

Blood alcohol levels
during crisis situations, 106-109
sampling procedures, 199-200

Body fluid monitoring, 199-200

Body language, of intervention team members, 143

Index

Documentation
  data collection and, 137-
  138
  during crisis situations,
  106-109
  post-intervention, 166,
  193-194
  as protection from
  subject's legal action,
  118-119
Double standards of health
professionals, 21-22
Drinking/using to feel
normal, 23, 28-29
Driving Under the
Influence (DUI) offenses,
88-90
"Dry drunk", 212

Early intervention,
importance of, 67
Education, of intervention
team members, 95-97
Ego strength, harmful
dependence and, 27-28
Emergency room staff, as
intervention data source,
82
Emotional continuum
  drinking/using to feel
  normal, 28-29
  harmful dependence, 27
  learning mood swing,
  24
  normal range, 23
  seeking mood swing,
  25-26
Emotional relapse, 212
Emotional syndrome of
chemical dependence, 23-
29, 34
Employee assistance
programs, 44

Employee Health Service,
as intervention data
source, 82, 84
Employer
  monitoring by, 190-192,
  207-208
  on intervention team,
  126
Employment applications,
as intervention data
source, 77
Enablers
  family members as, 36-
  39
  on intervention team,
  93-95, 129-130
  professional colleagues
  as, 35-36, 39-50
  self-inventory of, 50-51
Enabling behavior
  data collection retarded
  by, 49-50
  defined, 35-36
  denial or rationalization
  and, 1-2
  family/friends, 52
  institutional, 43-44, 52-
  53
  organizational, 41-43
  prescription writing as,
  46-47
  by professional
  colleagues, 3, 45-50, 52-
  53, 173
  suicide risk and, 163-
  164
  turned into assets, 162
Enzyme-Multiplied
Immunoassay Technique
(EMIT), 264
Enzyme immunoassay
(EIA), 264

Essential hypertension,
chemical dependence
indicator, 85
Ethical responsibilities,
chemical dependence and,
2-3
Evaluation, 181-183
  relapsed patients, 213-
  214
  subjects' refusal of,
  117-118
  written and oral
  summaries, 183
  written requests for, 141
Exclusion criteria for
intervention team, 93-95
Excuses from dependent
professional, during
intervention, 38, 115, 152
Expectations, outline of
during intervention, 161-
162
Extended family,
professional colleagues as,
39-50
Extended treatment, 219,
225-226
  recommendations for,
  186-187
Eye contact
  during intervention,
  143-144
  seating arrangements
  and, 150-151

Familial aspects of
chemical dependence, 12-
13
Families of dependent
professionals, 57-58
  closure procedures for,
  177-178, 180
  as enablers, 36-37, 52

284

When the Johnson Institute first opened its doors in 1966, few people knew or believed that alcoholism was a disease. Fewer still thought that anything could be done to help the chemically dependent person other than to wait for him or her to "hit bottom" and then pick up the pieces.

We've spent over twenty years spreading the good news that chemical dependence is a *treatable* disease. Through our publications, films, video and audiocassettes, and our training and consultation services, we've given hope and help to hundreds of thousands of people across the country and around the world. The intervention and treatment methods we've pioneered have restored shattered careers, healed relationships with co-workers and friends, saved lives, and brought families back together.

Today the Johnson Institute is an internationally recognized leader in the field of chemical dependence intervention, treatment, and recovery. Individuals, organizations, and businesses, large and small, rely on us to provide them with the tools they need. Schools, universities, hospitals, treatment centers, and other healthcare agencies look to us for experience, expertise, innovation, and results. With care, compassion, and commitment, we will continue to reach out to chemically dependent persons, their families, and the professionals who serve them.

To find out more about us, write or call:

7151 Metro Boulevard
Minneapolis, Mn 55435
1-800-231-5165
In MN: 1-800-247-0484
or 944-0511
In CAN: 1-800-447-6660

Need a copy for a friend? You may order directly.

TO CARE ENOUGH

Intervention with Chemically Dependent Colleagues
A Guide for Healthcare and Other Professionals

Linda R. Crosby, M.S.N., R.N. and LeClair Bissell, M.D., C.A.C.

A Johnson Institute Professional Series Book

$24.95

Order Form

Please send _____ copy (copies) of **TO CARE ENOUGH.** Price $24.95 per copy.
Please add $3.00 shipping for the first book and $1.25 for each additional copy.

Name (please print)

Address

City/State/Zip

Attention

Please note that orders under $75.00 must be prepaid.
If paying by credit card, please
complete the following:

☐ Bill the full payment to my credit card.

☐ VISA ☐ MasterCard ☐ American Express

Credit card number: _____

For MASTERCARD
Write the 4 digits below the account number: _____

Expiration date: _____

Signature on card: _____

For faster service, call
our Order Department
TOLL-FREE:
1-800-231-5165
In Minnesota call:
1-800-247-0484
or **(612) 944-0511**
In Canada call:
1-800-447-6660

Return this order form to: The Johnson Institute
                               7151 Metro Boulevard
                               Minneapolis, MN 55435-3425
Ship to (if different from above):

Name (please print)

Address

City/State/Zip